Cocoon of Love®

for

Cancer Caregivers

Get Through the Tough Times

ALSO BY SUSAN BROWNELL

Cocoon of Love® for Caregivers
365 Inspirational Readings for Busy Caregivers

Cocoon of Love®

for
Cancer Caregivers

Get Through the Tough Times

Susan Brownell

Current Edition:
This book is the second in a series of books titled "Cocoon of Love®"

DISCLAIMER:

This book is intended to offer inspirational support and encouragement for caregivers. It is not intended to provide medical advice or take the place of advice or treatment from trained medical professionals. If you have health questions or concerns about yourself or the one in your care, you should seek professional medical care. The publisher and author disclaim all liability that may be the result of the use of or misuse of information contained within this book.

First Edition: October 2013
Second Edition: October 2015

ISBN: 978-1-940826-03-5

Published by:
SB Leeder Publishing
Sparta, Wisconsin 54656

Email: info@susanbrownell.com

Websites: SusanBrownell.com
                     SanctuaryForCancerCaregivers.com

Social Media: https://www.facebook.com/susan.brownell.35
                     https://twitter.com/SusanBrownell
                     Connect with me on YouTube

Printed in the United States of America
First Printing: October 2013
Second Printing: October 2015

Dedication

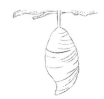

This book is lovingly dedicated to my mother, father, stepmother, and stepfather, who through their illness and dying taught me so much about caring and living.

Contents

Introduction

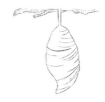

For the person with cancer, everything has suddenly changed. For those who love that person with cancer, the same is true. It can be a helpless and frustrating time in one's life. It can be a time of extreme sadness and soul-searching. A person with cancer handles the challenges of this disease in whatever ways possible to get by. The cancer patient deals with another day of chemotherapy and looks into the sad eyes of a loved one and wonders—wonders about the prognosis, wonders about the pain, wonders about the future.

The loved one caring for the cancer patient wonders too. The loved one wonders about having the ability to be an effective caregiver. The loved one wonders about having the strength to care and the knowledge to care. The loved one wonders about holding life together while traveling on this unknown path.

Emotions give way to new challenges. The cancer patient experiences a surge of emotions. The loved one giving care feels the impact of those emotions. At the same time, the caregiver is struggling with a wave of caregiver emotions. Caregivers to loved ones with cancer often feel inadequate, frightened, and alone. Some are angry at the cancer. Some are resentful. Many are sad. Many experience stress and feelings of helplessness. Caregivers want to make it better. It's a matter of wanting to do the right thing. Caregivers just aren't sure what that right thing is.

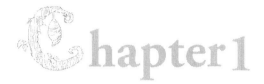

Chapter 1

C is for Cocoon

Love is all we have,
the only way that each can help the other.

~ Euripides ~

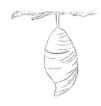

One word frees us of all the weight and pain of life.
That word is love.

~ Sophocles ~

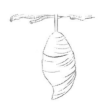

It's a word we've come to dread hearing. We hear it far too often. And when we hear it, we tend to associate it with a bad ending. The big "C". Cancer. Modern medicine has given us more options. Still the research continues. There are so many waiting and hoping for a cure for themselves or for loved ones. The debate continues over natural remedies versus traditional modern medicine. There are so many claims for herbal and natural remedies. There are other claims of various everyday items being touted as "The Cure". How does anyone begin to make a decision on treatment? And as progress continues, it just can't come fast enough for so many who are fighting the battle. It's something you wish no one would have to go through--especially, someone you love.

"I feel like I'm being surrounded with a cocoon of love," Mom told my stepdad. I'll never forget it. She lay in her hospital bed, newly diagnosed with terminal cancer, and only two weeks to live.

One by one, her seven children came home: one son from the East Coast, two sons from the West Coast, and all four daughters from Wisconsin. They all came to be with her, their dad, and stepdad, and with each other. They cried. They prayed. They desperately sought a reason for this. They consoled each other. They met with doctors and pastors. They came bearing gifts for their mom. They expressed their love in whatever ways they could. They bought her new nightgowns. They brought in her favorite country music. When she couldn't eat, they brought in things she normally loved: malts and her favorite candy bars. Her oldest son arrived in his Navy dress uniform because he knew she loved seeing him in uniform. They brought flowers. They rubbed her painful feet. They tenderly combed her hair. They told her they loved her. They left inspirational notes for her. They took turns holding her hand.

They had all-night vigils. Nothing seemed like enough. They saw her courage. They were in awe of her battle.

When she left, she gave them all a gift. She left them with the knowledge of the importance and power of love at life's most challenging times. She left them transformed by a cocoon of love, which they helped construct. They were not aware of how many more times they would have to use that gift in the years to come.

What gets you through the tough times in life? It's love. It's acts of kindness. Love comes in many forms. Can you ever have enough love? Where does the love come from? Sometimes it comes from within. It protects, it nourishes, it helps you grow and flourish in what would otherwise be unbearable times. Some of this love is from you to your loved one. Some of this love you must give to yourself. How do you find the time and the strength to give and receive this love when you are overwhelmed? You can learn from a beautiful example in nature—the butterfly.

Have you ever been to a butterfly garden? It's extraordinary. It's so uplifting and beautiful. It is a slice of heaven! Imagine a beautiful garden with birds, trickling waters, beautiful flowers, and an abundance of green shrubs and trees. On one tree, you notice a large caterpillar slowly eating his way up a leaf. Nearby you see another caterpillar looking so chubby he appears he could burst. As you look closely, you also see a chrysalis, often called a cocoon. As you look around, you notice many more in different stages of development. Some are newly formed and of various colors. Some have become transparent, meaning a butterfly is reaching maturity and will soon emerge. Some have butterflies emerging from them. Some of the butterflies are sitting fairly still and drying before they can fly. Some are starting to exercise their wings a bit. Some butterflies are already flying—swooping high, then low. Some land on flowers and leaves. Many flit about in an erratic pattern.

For so many living things that come into this world, you cannot watch their progress as they grow, develop, and come into this world. They are formed internally, within another living creature. Butterflies are quite different. Their entire life cycle happens out in this big world. If you are fortunate enough, you can watch the process in awe. It's much like when your loved one is diagnosed with cancer. You can watch that, too, in awe, and the changes it creates in them, and in yourself. It's a challenge. Sometimes you wonder how people get through it. But, as you watch, you soon see, there is a transformation taking place--one for your loved one, and one for you, their caregiver. As you look more closely, you soon see that the silk thread that holds the cocoon together is love. There are the threads of self-love to get you through this great challenge, and there are silk threads of love gently wrapping around your loved one with cancer.

Just as life is fragile, butterflies are very fragile. Most butterflies have a very short lifespan. Some butterflies may have injuries and have a shorter lifespan than most. Think of how fragile a butterfly is. When butterflies emerge from the cocoon, they do not know how long they will be of this world, but they go forth courageously and live their lives to the fullest.

Just as the caterpillar instinctively recognizes when it's time to construct a cocoon, so it is with cancer patients and their loved ones who care for them. You will soon realize that you and your loved one both need a cocoon to give you a chance to process what's happening. A cocoon will protect your loved one and yourself for a period of time until you have both reached a point of being able to move forward with the next steps. Your cocoon of love may mature before your loved one's cocoon. That's okay. The silk threads of love will know when it is time to loosen their hold on the cocoon.

*Caregiving is one of the most loving gifts
you can give someone.*

~ Susan Brownell ~

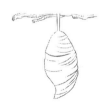

Chapter 2

The Need to Feed

After the diagnosis occurs, cancer caregivers and their loved ones have a voracious appetite for information. They feed on everything they can to gather up answers to their unending questions and to deal with their raw emotions.

~ Susan Brownell ~

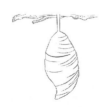

We live in the information age. Everywhere we look we see large screens with news. There are magazines available in print and electronically. You can buy, rent, or borrow DVDs on many subjects or watch educational programs on television. You can read on e-readers and do research on a tablet. When a loved one is diagnosed with cancer, you both want answers.

Sorting through all the information available, sometimes you have to decide if a source is trustworthy. Sometimes you have to decide if the source of the information is only looking out for the welfare of their pocketbook. This makes the whole situation very emotional and challenging. This also presents opportunities for people to be taken advantage of both physically and financially. Advertising knows how to play with people's emotions. It is difficult to think clearly when you are dealing with all that you are.

Slow down, caregivers! Take a deep breath and relax. These things will be revealed to you, in time. So often, people imagine the worse. All too often they jump to some conclusions. More than likely, your loved one's team of doctors is still assembling more information to completely assess the situation. Take it one step at a time. This is a process.

At a time of life when he should have been enjoying himself, Dad had just been diagnosed with colon cancer. He was going to have surgery. This was totally unexpected. Everything was about to change. The emotions were incredible and the information too much to process. We had no clue of how to handle it. We knew this was not good news, but we really weren't sure what we were dealing with. One thing we did know. We were scared. No, we were terrified.

I really didn't know my dad very well. He and my mom divorced when I was four and my brother was one. My brother and I would travel to visit him and my stepmother for two weeks every summer and one week over the Christmas holidays.

He was a semi driver and worked long hours. He had a great sense of humor and was constantly playing jokes on his buddies. He was well-known and well-liked about town. Before the cancer, he had a heart attack, but he recovered and returned to trucking. After he "retired", he took on three part-time jobs. He loved to work, and he loved to be out around people. He never came across as mushy or overly emotional. He just loved being around people. He loved to have fun.

After I married, I was busy with work, my husband, and raising two children. We would go to visit my dad and stepmother a couple of times a year. He lived two and a half hours away. They would come to see us about once a year. I was horrified to think that I could lose him and had never really gotten to know him. Guilt overcame me. Why hadn't I made a greater effort to spend more time with him as an adult? If he passed away, would his grandchildren have many memories of him?

Everyone I had ever known with cancer had passed away with one exception. My mother-in-law had survived breast cancer after undergoing a radical mastectomy and radiation treatments about fifteen years earlier. I was so thankful for her recovery, as I love her dearly. Meanwhile, I felt like my dad had just received a death sentence. I felt powerless, guilty, sad, and angry all at once.

You and your loved one are still reeling from the shock of the diagnosis. You are both experiencing an emotional tsunami wave. Your mind is trying to process many things. Your initial thoughts may revolve around fear. There is fear for your loved one's well-being. There is fear for you. There may be a fear of caregiving.

You start asking yourself questions. How will your loved one's life change? Can you handle it? How will your life change? How will you find out about all the medical stuff? How will the rest of the family deal with this? Where will the money come from to pay all the medical bills? Who will be able to take the loved one in for treatments if needed? Will anyone else be willing to help, or will you have to do this alone? Will your loved one be able to work again? Will your loved one survive this illness?

Feelings start to surface very quickly. You may feel vulnerable and inadequate. Yes, you may even feel a bit of resentment. Feelings of resentment often lead to a feeling of guilt. Some cancer caregivers feel anger.

It all seems like too much to deal with. You and your loved one need to have time to figure this out and deal with it. Everything is moving fast, and you and your loved one are having trouble keeping up. As you both realize you need a cocoon, you also realize you're going to have to build your cocoons.

Just as the caterpillar feeds voraciously in preparation for weaving a cocoon, so it is with you and your loved one. The caregiver and the loved one with cancer feed on the situation and available information. You take in all the calories you can, as you'll need to digest this in-depth shortly.

You feed on immense amounts of information, sandwiched between some very strong emotions. You search out answers to countless questions with an appetite that knows no limit. You and your loved one are on a fact-finding mission to help prepare yourselves for what lies ahead. Your insatiable appetites for information are helping you prepare for the construction of your cocoons, so you can begin to process the information and make important decisions.

You and your loved one gather your information, most of which will be processed later, when you are in your cocoons. There are many pieces of information you will need to gather.

Many hospitals and clinics now have a Patient Navigator to help you get through the medical network. These are certainly available at larger clinics and hospitals. If your hospital does not have one, ask them to refer you to someone working there who can help you navigate your way through their medical system.

Find a support system for you and your loved one. Lean on your best friends. Get help from your family. If you belong to clubs or social groups, make people aware of what you are dealing with. Someone may step forward to help you. If you are involved in a church or religious organization, make people aware of your situation. Often they have committees to help care for their members. Many times caring individuals will step forward with an offer to help. These individuals can be a source of comfort and encouragement during the difficult days that lie ahead. Check for organizations consisting of volunteers to help with specific tasks. Check with social workers, clinics, hospitals, county agencies, and volunteer groups, such as Faith in Action. These organizations are available to help with a great variety of things, including grocery shopping, transportation, teaching individuals how to use email, and many other helpful everyday functions. Take advantage of this opportunity.

You need support to provide you with information, inspiration, encouragement, and a network of resources. With the demands of caregiving and your daily life, you don't have time to go to a lot of meetings. You need to keep it simple and have information easily available at any hour of the day. You never know when the next crisis will occur. You never know how many hours a day a loved one will need your assistance. You need flexibility. Online support offers information specifically designed to help those who care for a loved one with cancer. Nurses' hotlines can also be very beneficial.

Just as a cocoon provides a form of protection as the caterpillar turns into a butterfly, caregivers feel a need to protect their loved one who has cancer. How will you protect them? Your loved one may or may not be ready to deal with others right away. You'll need to try to find out their feelings about that. Some well-intentioned people may say the wrong thing. Your loved one may not be quite ready to hear all the details for a while. You need to allow them time to process, rest, think, and recuperate. You need to honor their wishes as best you can.

At the same time, you may feel a need to protect yourself. How will you hold down your fear and stress? How will you "be there" for your loved one while you may be feeling panic-stricken? How will you get enough rest when you know you'll have many extra duties to take on? How can you quickly and easily gather up what you need to know to be prepared and be able to deal with this?

What will be your filter? In these days of information overload, sometimes there is too much information to sift through to locate what you really need. Find a few good, reliable sources to follow to reduce the time needed to search the Internet. Check for support resources at your loved one's clinic or hospital. Some provide a resource library, where you may be able to check a book out and learn more about your loved one's illness. Some provide free samples of magazines for cancer patients and their caregivers. Some of these magazines have coupons inside offering a free subscription for cancer patients or their caregivers.

Slow down the pace of your lives while you prepare to process what is happening. Have a family member screen your calls and your loved one's calls. Focus on just what you have to for a period of time so that you have more time to process the information. This can consume a lot of energy, so save yourself for it in any way you can.

After you and your loved one have gathered up some information and had some time to digest it, you will move on to the next step.

It is time to determine the game plan for your loved one. How will you accomplish the physical care of the loved one? Will you need help to take care of your loved one? Is there a family member, friend, or neighbor available to help with your loved one's needs, care, and support? If it becomes necessary to have in-home care, can you get help with that? How will you accomplish the emotional care of the loved one? Who and what have been a source of emotional encouragement for your loved one in the past? Are those things available now as a means of emotional encouragement? What new things could you add as a source of emotional encouragement for your loved one? How will you find out your loved one's wishes? What will the costs of care be? At this point it is easy to focus totally on your loved one.

There is one more important area that needs your attention. Now is also the time to implement the game plan for you. How will you accomplish the physical care for yourself? How will you accomplish the emotional care for yourself? Do you have any special health care needs? What do you do for yourself now to maintain good health? How can you continue to do those things for yourself in the challenging days ahead? How will the rest of the family function? When you are otherwise occupied during the demanding days to come, who will help and support you?

You could compare this process to building a house. First you gather up a lot of information. Then you have to look all of that over and analyze it. It can be very overwhelming. You know you will have to make a lot of decisions. Your head hurts as you try to process it. You need to treat this as you would any big project. Get the big picture first. Know what your end result goal is—realistically. Design a blueprint. Then go backwards and make the little decisions that realistically support that end result. Chunk it down. This takes place after you are in the cocoon stage analyzing. If your loved one is seriously ill and possibly terminal, you may not know that right away. Your incoming information is in chunks too. You often won't get the entire picture immediately.

As the caterpillar's girth expands from consuming all that it has, it becomes obvious that construction time is near. The feasting winds down, in preparation for the weaving of the cocoon. Soon the caterpillars will be surrounded by a safe, secure cocoon.

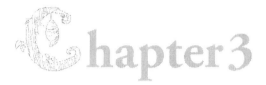

Extreme Cocoon Construction

Being a caregiver is hard work. Entering the cancer caregiver experience for the first time is like being hired as a construction worker with no skills. You put on your hard hat. You grab a few power tools. You watch the other more skilled workers and hope you can build this house without it falling down.

~ Susan Brownell ~

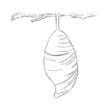

*Give your labor as an extension of a compassionate,
loving heart.*

~ Susan Brownell ~

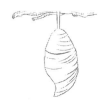

Being a caregiver is hard work! It's physically and mentally exhausting. You are continuously pulled in many directions at once. You are forced to make difficult decisions when time and resources do not allow you to accomplish everything you feel you must do. And under all of it, there's a great deal of emotion. Emotions can be exhausting too. You need time to pull back, examine the situation, and get a plan together. It's important that you build your cocoon now so you can find the space to deal with what is to come.

Just like any good construction crew, you select a good building site for your cocoon. Pick a quiet place. Choose a place where you can find solace and peace. That's not an easy thing with all the turbulence in your life right now. It is, however, important. Where will you find your quiet place? Will it be outdoors? In a park? On a favorite walking trail? Or will it be in a room in your house that's known to be your space?

You gather your materials. Although construction crews may have a highly detailed and technical floor plan, you do not. You have no formal instructions on how to build your cocoon. This may cause alarm and make you feel inadequate. You may even start to panic.

How do you do it? How do you build your cocoon? You've never built one before. Think about that fattened-up caterpillar getting ready to make a cocoon. Has the caterpillar made a cocoon before? No, but he still is able to get the task done. Have you ever cared for a loved one with cancer before? Perhaps not, but you can do it. The caterpillar trusts its instincts to guide it in the cocoon-building process. You, the caregiver, will have certain instincts that will help you also. You also have help and resources available to you. Use your instincts to tap into those valuable and helpful resources. Now is not the time to be a one-person show!

The process begins. The caterpillar firmly attaches itself to the twig that will be its home during the transformation. The caterpillar begins weaving the cocoon and spinning the silk or golden threads.

You also spin a cocoon of silk threads to protect yourself and give yourself some "away" time to process this major change in your life. Simultaneously, your loved one begins to spin his cocoon. It is possible that as a caregiver, you may have to lovingly provide some gentle help to your loved one with his cocoon.

Weaving and spinning, twisting and turning, wriggling and covering are all part of the procedures. The caterpillar quiets himself as he covers the last of his body with the silky, golden threads that put the finishing touches on the cocoon. And then…there's silence and stillness.

The building of a cocoon is rather fascinating. What's happening inside the cocoon? There is a miraculous metamorphosis of you, the caregiver, and your loved one with cancer. At last, you and your loved one are able to retreat to process the diagnosis, prognosis, and the vast amount of information you have received. At last, you will be able to think about what this means to you and your loved one. Finally, you have an opportunity for some quiet time to digest that big feast your caterpillar just consumed.

As you prepare for your metamorphosis within the cocoon, you and your loved one must establish some basic things. Consider what you've lost. Consider what you still have. Let go of things that don't matter. Cleanse yourself of negative feelings, such as hatred, jealousy, competition. Leave behind you: enemies, family feuds, coveting, bitterness, and anger. Conserve your energy to focus on the tasks at hand. Think about what is most important in life and what is most important right now. Don't expect a cookie-cutter response from your loved one or yourself. It's a different emotional journey for each cancer patient and each caregiver. Not everyone processes and handles the news the same way. Everyone is different. Every situation is different. Everyone must respond as to what is appropriate for themselves.

Now that your cocoon is constructed, quiet time is in effect.

Quiet time for your loved one— there are many decisions to make. Quiet time for you—time to think, time to process, time to analyze, time to prioritize, time to purge yourself of toxic negative emotions and to be positive, time to make a difference for you and for them. You must come up with a plan to help get you and your loved one through this. With so much activity after the diagnosis, you and your loved one now need quiet time. Silence is good for the soul— your soul and theirs. Get into the moment. Close out all the noise of daily life. Eliminate the continuous chatter of television, radio, and electronic media. Experience the silence so that you, too, can eventually touch a soul.

We need to find God, and he cannot be found in noise and restlessness.
God is the friend of silence.
See how nature – trees, flowers, grass – grows in silence;
see the stars, the moon, and the sun, how they move in silence…
We need silence to be able to touch souls.

~ Mother Teresa ~

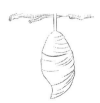

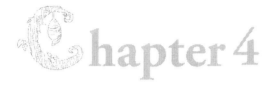

Chapter 4

Cocoon Care for Them: Surround Them with Love

A caregiver's tears of love mean nothing
if he turns away when his loved one needs him most.

~ Susan Brownell ~

I can do all things through him who strengthens me.

~ Philippians 4:13 ~

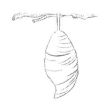

Your loved one goes through several phases on this journey. Often he begins the journey with denial. It is easier to live in denial of what is happening. He may follow the denial with anger, and who could blame him? Eventually he reaches a point of acceptance. Finally, he will reach a point of resignation, that he can finally act on the acceptance. There is no timetable on when or how long it takes the person with cancer to reach each phase. Sometimes a loved one may revert back to the anger phase. It can vary immensely. The details and timing of this journey are not the same for loved ones with cancer or their caregivers, but all have some things in common. Caregivers may or may not reach acceptance before their loved one. The important thing is to be aware of what the mindset is of your loved one and yourself and respond accordingly.

This is one of those times when it is awkward for some people. You feel terrible about what is happening to your loved one. You want to show your love, but you aren't sure how. You know he is still grappling with how to process and handle his situation. You listen and watch for signals. You learn to read your loved one. You hope you are getting it right.

Then came more cancer—part two of two bouts of it. We all knew it was not good. I couldn't bear the thought of losing my dad when I had spent so little time with him. I lived 130 miles from him. I drove to see him every other weekend for much of his illness. It was so hard to see him deteriorate before my eyes. I didn't know how to act. I didn't want to let him see my sadness, so I made every effort to be upbeat when I was around him. I felt rather fake for being that way. But I could see he needed cheering up. He had lost his voice from an experimental cancer treatment during his first bout of cancer. He could only speak in a whisper. During his illness, we probably had more whispering conversations than voice conversations all those other years combined. When it was hard to find something to talk about, we talked about old memories, fun times, and some of the many practical jokes he played on people.

Dad was losing weight and getting weaker. He seemed quieter than before, and frail. He didn't complain about his lot in life, but it was obvious, life was never to be the same for him again.

My stepmother told me how Dad's spirits were always better for many days after I had been there. All this time, I thought my visits were so powerless, and yet, they were helping him much more than I knew.

I was continuously amazed at what was important to Dad during those last months. I tried to listen intently and go along with whatever he wanted to do at that time. One weekend he wanted to take a drive in the country to see his birthplace and where he was raised. It was like he was saying his goodbyes, and he wanted his daughter to know some of these things. It was heartwarming, in a bittersweet way.

During several visits he brought up his concerns about his "Hayshaker Girls" movie. Dad was an avid citizens Band Radio participant. He loved talking on his Citizens Band Radio to truckers and members of various CB clubs. His CB handle was "Hayshaker". No doubt, it was reminiscent of his days of farming when he was much younger.

In keeping with his love of joking around, he had dared a group of men to dress up in some dresses and bunny-type outfits. He dared them to do a chorus line dance at an annual town event one summer wearing those clothes. Amazingly, he got some takers! The group of big, burly men surprised him in their form-fitting girly clothes, bursting forth with hairy chests and legs. They performed a chorus line dance like none other. Someone filmed it using the old-style reel-to-reel movie camera. On the film, Dad was caught by surprise and can be seen laughing until the tears roll down his face. He had to take his glasses off to wipe away the tears of laughter. He proudly got out the reel of film, so he could play it for me. He was weak and off-balance as he set up the heavy projector. I worried he'd drop it on his slipper-covered feet. I worried he'd tip over and fall down because he was so weak and tipsy. I'd heard the story many times and seen the pictures, but I'd never seen the movie before. It was hilarious! Dad thought the days of the reel-to-reel cameras were long over and that someday no one would be able to watch the film that he treasured. It so captured his personality and love of playing pranks. I knew he was looking for a solution as it came up every weekend I was there. One weekend, I brought my camcorder. Having no video camera skills, I had no idea how to do this. I had Dad run the movie, and I recorded the images as they were projected onto the movie screen. Today's video gurus would laugh at the thought of such a method. I was amazed to play back the videotape and see that it actually worked! Dad was pleased that his infamous Hayshaker Girls would now be preserved for future generations. Many might feel it was silly to make such a big production out of this movie. It was very important to Dad that this warm memory of him live on. It was one of those little things that some cancer patients just feel a need to do.

Some types of insects undergo the transformation process in a chrysalis, rather than a cocoon, but the concept is the same. For example, a monarch butterfly technically is transformed within a green chrysalis. A moth typically is transformed within a white or brown cocoon. Both a chrysalis and a cocoon house the pupa as it is transformed. Since most people commonly refer to a cocoon rather than a chrysalis when speaking of this process, we will refer to a cocoon instead of a chrysalis throughout this book.

The butterfly cocoon is self-contained and self-regulated. The butterfly cocoon acts as a protective casing. Contained within the cocoon is the pupa. The pupa is the undeveloped butterfly in a non-feeding stage. Over a period of time, the pupa slowly transforms into a butterfly. For a good deal of the time, you cannot see inside the cocoon, but as the metamorphosis continues, some cocoons become transparent. The monarch butterfly provides an example of that. At that time, without disturbing it, you can peek inside for a glimpse of the transformation taking place.

You and your loved one are slowly transforming also. You are both adjusting to a new life with new challenges and perhaps a shift in responsibilities.

Imagine how your loved one must feel. Perhaps your loved one is on an extended leave from work because of his illness. Perhaps he is depressed. You see a big change in his personality.

Perhaps he can no longer do the things he did before the illness struck. Perhaps he is so sick, he can do nothing. Perhaps he has had to give up working or driving. Perhaps there is little to no hope for a good outcome from the treatment. That would be devastating news. You can imagine how your loved one feels, but you can't really know how they feel. One thing is certain. Your loved one could use some cocoon care.

One of the best things you can do for your loved one during this difficult time is to give him your love. You wish you could do so much more. You feel this is so little to offer at such a difficult time.

Can your loved one feel the love they are given? Yes—more than you know! So, pour it on. Surround him with love. But how can you do this? The main need of your loved one is basic. Be there for them. Don't turn away. Just be there. You will be amazed at how many ways there are to show your love during this unbelievably difficult time.

See how many of the following ways you can show some cocoon care and love to your loved one:

- Verbalize your love.

- Be the catalyst to help others verbalize and show their love.

- Arrange for home care, if they need it, or if you need it for your own sake.

- Provide hands-on caregiving if you are able.

- Research the support offered through hospice, if your loved one's prognosis is terminal.

- Help your loved one with pain management. That is not to say you should play doctor. You do need to educate yourself to a certain extent on pain management. Ask your loved one's medical professionals for some brochures or books on pain management. If your loved one is on hospice, they will be an invaluable source of help to you when dealing with pain management for your loved one. At times, your loved one may be too "out of it" to keep track of medication times, so you may need to assist him with getting organized with that. You or someone else may need to see to it that your loved one takes pain medications at the appropriate time. This also applies to getting prescriptions refilled. Establish a plan to monitor when it is time to refill the pain medications, so you can ensure they are refilled before running out. If pain gets out of control because of being overdue for a dose of medication, it is sometimes more difficult to get it back under control again. You may need to help by communicating with the doctor or nurse if you feel the current medications aren't controlling the pain to an acceptable level. They will determine if changes need to be made to current medications. Never assume the role of deciding if you should increase doses of pain medications. Granted, it is very difficult to see your loved one in pain, but only a medical professional should make decisions on increasing a dosage or the frequency of taking medications. It is very dangerous for non-medical professionals to take this matter into their own hands. Never hesitate to contact your loved one's medical team if you feel a change is needed. Your loved one may not be able to verbalize his need or even recognize his need for pain management.

- Become more aware of habits, food dislikes, eating habits, new health concerns, personality changes. Your loved one isn't feeling well. You can't count on him to inform the doctors of these changes. When people aren't feeling well or in denial of the seriousness of their illness, they may not want to acknowledge some of these issues. Sometimes the caregiver must make the loved one's medical team aware of changes. This can help them in their overall treatment plan.

- Watch for signs of depression, which happens often to loved ones with cancer. His doctor is used to treating this depression due to the illness with medication or counseling.

- Coordinate spiritual care for your loved one, if this is desired. Remember, if your loved one isn't feeling well, any little coordination or tasks you can relieve him of, will help lessen the great weight he feels at this time. Remember also, if your loved one has a condition that is continuously deteriorating, you will want to take care of things like this while your loved one is still conscious and coherent and can process the information and make decisions. For many loved ones with cancer, this can make all the difference in finding peace. We will discuss this more in-depth later.

• Send or give your loved one inspirational messages and cards via the post office, email, in person, in his lunch box, or hidden throughout the house in places your loved one will find them.

• When words fail you…just be there.

• When words fail you…hold your loved one's hand.

• When words fail you…hug your loved one.

• When words fail you…tenderly kiss your loved one's forehead.

• Show some empathy.

• Watch and listen.

• Try to make it easy for him to communicate…early on and until the end, if he is terminal. It is often said that the sense of hearing is one of the last things to stop working. Your loved one may be able to hear you but not respond. Maybe he would like to interact with you in some small way as death draws near. Perhaps you have a message to share with him and you want to ensure he hears it. Perhaps you are trying to find out if he has pain or would like something done for him. You could ask him a yes or no question and ask him to squeeze your hand once if the answer is yes. When he becomes too weak to squeeze your hand, you could ask him a yes or no question and tell him to blink his eyes once for yes or twice for no. It is also important to keep in mind that you should be mindful of any conversations you have in his presence. Even though your loved one may appear to be completely unable to communicate, you should assume he may be hearing everything that is said in his presence. This may mean that some sensitive conversations need to occur away from his room.

- Respect his wishes, in love, if you can. Of course, you will take into consideration such things as his safety and well-being as you respect his wishes.

- Help others to respect his wishes, in love.

- Savor your time together.

- Don't always have a gray cloud hanging over you. One of your biggest challenges as a caregiver is to find a balance when dealing with your loved one. You want to be upbeat and encouraging to your loved one. However, if the prognosis is bad, you sometimes need to be real too. Your loved one needs to know that you do understand the seriousness of the situation. Offering to listen to him and his feelings can help overcome some of this.

- Be real. Sometimes you will show your real emotions. Sometimes you may cry in front of him.

- Be accepting of your loved one. You may see personality changes. Your loved one may be concerned if you will still love them.

After my mother-in-law had a radical mastectomy, she had radiation treatments. She told me how her skin in that area had turned dry and black. Just hearing about it made me uncomfortable. Whenever she would discuss it with me, she would say, "You can see it if you want to." Every time she brought it up, I would tell her, "No, that's okay." She just kept bringing it up. I finally realized that she wanted me to see her disfigured body so she could see my reaction to it. The next time she asked if I would like to see her disfigured area, I said that I would.

She removed her top and showed me the entire surgical area and the black area. I did my best to not look shocked. We discussed it a bit, and that was the end of it. She needed to know that she was accepted as she was and that I would not look away in shock and disgust.

- You may find your loved one's emotions vary immensely. This is all part of the journey. Although this is not always easy, try to not take offense at things your loved one says. Your loved one is under a lot of stress, may not be feeling well, and is experiencing a lot of emotion, which fluctuates regularly.

During his illness, I saw my stepfather cry, which I had never seen before. Suddenly life became very emotional for him. It was difficult to see this man, who was formerly in control of his emotions, become so emotional.

My father sometimes got grumpy, which I had never seen before. He would sometimes sit in a chair all day. He would vomit daily—often several times. He had little appetite, so he became weak. What I didn't know at the time was that the medications affected the way foods tasted. He eventually became so ill and weak that he had to quit working. He used to live to work. Giving up working was a major life change for him. My stepmother complained that he did nothing all day when she was gone to work. What she failed to understand was that he didn't feel good enough to do anything. Because of his illness and inability to work, he became depressed, which also caused him to not do things he used to do.

There are many things that you can do to help your loved one get his mind on other things. Even though your loved one may feel badly, an enjoyable distraction can work wonders. It may temporarily get his mind off how poorly he feels or the results of that last blood test that came back from the lab today. Of course, you will have to consider his current condition as you look at these options. Think about things your loved one used to enjoy. Think about new things your loved one may want to do, as well. At first it may seem like nothing is really appropriate, so you may need to push yourself to see some possibilities. Here are some ideas to help you get started:

- Put up a bird feeder near a window, porch, or sunroom for him to watch the birds. If your loved one is feeling well enough, you could even have him feed the birds.

- Put up a bird bath. Many people enjoy watching the birds come and go to bathe and drink from the bird bath. Put it near a window, so your loved one can watch it from inside the house. Put a water dripper in the bird bath. This will draw much more traffic to the bird bath.

- Put a heater in your bird bath during the winter. There's not much going on at that time of year. A heated bird bath will draw lots of activity, which will provide your loved one with something to help pass the time at a time of year that holds special challenges.

- Provide a bird identification book to help keep your loved one occupied as he watches the bird feeder and bird bath.

- Put a small tabletop water fountain in the house near where your loved one likes to sit. Listening to the peaceful water flow can provide some stress relief.

- Get some stress-reducing CDs for your loved one to listen to. Some may have subliminal messages to calm the listener. Some provide ocean sounds, brook sounds, birds by the ocean sounds, and various other nature sounds. These are often available in discount stores, department stores, and online. Some are even specifically made for people with health problems.

- Get out some old family videos or home movies. View these together.

- Make new videos, especially of special days and family get-togethers. Create new memories for your loved one and the entire family.

- Plan family reunions so that your loved one can see relatives. Some people stay away after relatives are diagnosed with cancer. Some feel uncomfortable and don't know what to say. This is even truer if the loved one is terminal. Sometimes people are more comfortable visiting when the caregiver or another person is present. If some family members can't attend, ask them to send photos, or write about some family stories they would like to share.

- Get out some of your loved one's old family photo albums. Look at them together, slowly over a period of time. Ask a lot of questions. This often can help get his mind off things if he is not feeling well. There's probably a lot of family history that you aren't even aware of. Most people love to talk about years back and share nostalgic stories with anyone who is interested.

- Try using music therapy. This can help calm and mentally transport cancer patients to a better place. Collections of music assembled for just this purpose are available online and in bookstores.

- Help your loved one join an online support group for cancer patients to interact with each other and support each other. The cancer patient can share tips and feelings with others. He can vent to others without judgment. He can vent to others without fear of upsetting family members and those closest to him. He can gain new friends and support from others who understand what he is dealing with. Sometimes a cancer patient may not want to discuss something with family and friends; however, he may wish to discuss it with a stranger or someone in the support group.

- Bring your loved one little gifts. These don't have to be expensive. For example, bring a favorite treat he likes, a book, or a knick-knack. If there's something that's hard to talk about, you could give him an inspirational card or a book that addresses what you can't find the words to say. That may help open the door to the conversation you would like to have with him. After some time, ask if he read the book and what he thought about it. If your loved one doesn't feel up to reading, perhaps an audio book would be the best solution.

- Give or mail an inspirational card each day or every other day that you can't be with your loved one. It reminds him that you are thinking of him. These cards can be homemade, store-bought, or electronic to be delivered via email. The e-card sites can provide animated, musical, or just plain text and image messages. These can be inspirational, cheerful, and downright funny. On some of the electronic sites, the e-cards can be set up some time in advance with a designated mail-out date. This helps the cancer patient feel they are being thought of regularly, while freeing the caregiver of having to set these up every day. Some e-cards are free, and some are a paid service at a reasonable price for a one- or two-year subscription. If you do a search on the Internet for "e-cards" you will retrieve a list of many of these sites.

- Help your loved one enjoy the blessings of children and grandchildren, as applicable.

◻ If your loved one has children and grandchildren nearby, encourage them to visit regularly.

◻ When children or grandchildren can't visit as often as you'd like, have them make videos to send your loved one.

◻ If there are no children or grandchildren, consider interaction with nieces and nephews, if they are close to your loved one.

◻ Use one of the live video-conferencing methods available using your computer or television, if you have a smart TV. It will allow your loved one to see and talk to friends and relatives on his terms, from the comfort of his home when he feels up to it. Your loved one could even appear on camera in his pajamas! This is great if your loved one is weak or not feeling well. Treat it as a come-as-you-are visit. Maybe the caller could be in pajamas too! There is no need to dress up or schedule time ahead, unless you want the caller to check with you first to see if your loved one is up to visiting. You can visit live with two-way video and audio. If money is a factor, there are no long-distance charges for some of these services. Your loved one may not feel up to struggling with the technical aspect of this, so you may want to make yourself available to help him place the calls, especially the first few times. Make a reference sheet with step-by-step instructions. To make the instructions even more helpful, you could insert screen captures of the step-by-step directions into the Reference Sheet.

¤ Get a digital picture frame and put a digital slide show in it. Your loved one will be able to sit and look at pictures of happier times. Be careful to not get one that is too small if your loved one is older. A digital picture frame that displays an 8-by-10-inch-size photo works well. Include old photos of family members, friends, fun times over the years, and special events. This can be done by scanning the old photos to use with the digital picture frame. If you don't own a high-quality scanner, check your local large chain discount store or large chain pharmacy. They usually have good quality scanners. Use of a digital picture frame is a great tool for those who spend most of their day sitting in a chair. Set the frame up close to and facing the chair your loved one usually sits in, so when nothing else seems doable, all it takes is looking that direction to enjoy the pictures. Drive around his town and take photos of familiar places so when he is feeling very confined, he can at least see his old familiar places. Include all the seasons, or rotate groups of pictures so that he is seeing the current season's pictures now until the season changes. You can set these frames to turn on and off at a specific time of day. You can adjust the settings and the frequency of the changing of the photos. Some also play movies and music as well. The movie feature is nice if your loved one is not able to attend special family events. If your loved one has television in the same room, you might want to keep it simple and simply do photos without music or movies.

¤ Similar to how you would use a digital picture display, be sure your loved one has framed print photos of those most important in his life on display in the rooms where he spends most of his time. If your loved one is elderly, be sure the photos are large enough for him to see. Also, place the photos close enough for him to see from his favorite chair.

- Help your loved one enjoy the blessings of animals and pets.

  ¤ The love of a pet brings a special comfort. They are so accepting. They seem to sense when people are ill. They also are great company and are certain to provide some laughs. My stepmother never liked cats. Much to my surprise, after my dad passed away, she got a cat when she was ill. She found she liked the company of the cat. As you consider contact with pets, be sure your loved one isn't suffering from a compromised immune system or allergies. You may need to check with his doctor.

  ¤ If there is no pet in your loved one's life, how about some "doggy therapy"? For example, some people take their dogs to nursing homes and hospitals as therapy dogs. Perhaps you could get one to visit your loved one once or twice a week. Another option might be to take your pet or a friend's pet to your loved one's house, if you are not a live-in caregiver.

  ¤ Provide your loved one with animal videos to watch. Dogs and cats, especially, can be very entertaining. There are lots of humorous ones available. There are several TV shows that often feature animal videos. You could even record these shows regularly to have them available for your loved one when he needs something to make him laugh. There are also many animal videos on the Internet. You may even have some homemade videos of your pets or your loved one's pets. You can also purchase videos. Since my dad was a bird lover, I gave him a video of birds. It had close-ups of birds in trees and at the bird bath. You could hear the birds' songs. This type of video makes people feel like they are outside. It really helps with cabin fever during the winter. Also, it can be very relaxing.

¤   If your loved one uses a computer, email him inspirational quotes. Email him links to funny or inspirational videos on the Internet.

• Help your loved one enjoy the blessings of nature. There is so much beauty outside. There is something very therapeutic about enjoying a walk in the woods, a stroll in the park, or sitting on a park bench on a beautiful morning, if your loved one is up to the physical aspects of this.

• You probably don't know everything there is to know about your loved one and his family. Now is the time to get to know him better. Show an interest in your loved one's family history. Most people love to talk about their family history and share things about their growing-up years. Ask about the "old days." Ask about his fondest memories of childhood and school, work, friends, pets, hobbies, vacations, and holidays. Find out about family ancestors you never really got to know. Inquire about life events. Ask what he thinks about timely topics. You might be amazed at some of the things you learn about your loved one that you may have never known about!

- Plan a special project together, if your loved one is up to it. What are some things that the two of you like to do? Does your loved one have a special skill you'd like to learn? Do you have a special skill your loved one would like to learn? Most people love to share their knowledge with others or do a project with a family member. This could be spread over a period of time. When your loved one feels good, you can work on it. When your loved one is under the weather, just wait a while until he is feeling better. Sometimes he may feel under the weather, but just need to focus on something to get his mind off it. Getting him involved in something he enjoys will help get his mind off how he feels. Here are some ideas:

  ◻ Learn to bake an apple pie.

  ◻ Learn to knit.

  ◻ Learn to quilt.

  ◻ Learn to do woodworking with electrical tools.

  ◻ Learn to do wood carvings by hand.

  ◻ Learn to paint.

  ◻ Learn to play guitar or piano.

  ◻ Write a family memoir.

  ◻ Write some poetry.

  ◻ Put together a family scrapbook or photo album.

- Do research and put together a family tree.

- Go fishing.

- Go hunting.

- Go walking or bicycling, if your loved one is capable.

- Do online shopping.

- Do online or in-person auctions.

- Go to yard sales.

- Research antiques online.

- Research the family tree online.

- Visit the library and borrow books.

- Play online games or games on phones and tablets, or video games.

- Start or continue a collection of coins, stamps, buttons, glassware, or information about specific topics. If your loved one isn't up to leaving home to look for items, consider Internet shopping.

- Play board games, such as chess, checkers, Monopoly®, or Scrabble®. These games could be left set-up and continued as your loved one feels able to participate.

- Play card games. Your loved one may not feel well enough to deal with learning a new card game or board game. Ask what the old favorites are and try to stay with something familiar or easy, if that is a concern. If you need an easy game to play, try one of the children's card games, such as Go Fish. The goal is to get your loved one to focus on something other than how badly he feels at the moment.

- Work a giant jigsaw puzzle. This can be done over a period of time. Set up a special table for the puzzle and work on it as it fits into the schedule.

- Do Sudoku puzzles.

- Do crossword puzzles.

- Fill out word game books.

- Together, make up a trivia game about the family. This would be great fun at the next family gathering.

- Write a family history.

- Take up photography—even from the car window as you do rides in the car!

- Make a video diary. This could be about what your loved one is doing, about the journey of his illness, about his love of family, his biography, a hobby, or any number of things.

◻ Start a gratitude journal. Help your loved one focus on the positives in his life rather than dwelling on the negative. What happens each day that he is thankful for? For example: I am thankful for the door attendant at the clinic helping me today. I am thankful that a near car accident was avoided. I am thankful that I was able to eat a good meal today.

- Get one of the soothing sound players that you can set on ocean, brook, or gentle rain, to have playing in the background if your loved one has trouble sleeping. It will act as a relaxation device.

- Give freely of your time. Be available, but don't smother your loved one.

- Listen to your loved one. Look inside his heart. Watch for subtle clues.

- Communicate. Ask what he does and doesn't want. What helps? What doesn't? Are there people he really would like to see? Are there people who upset him that he would rather not see at this time when he just isn't feeling up to coping with extra drama?

- Call and encourage your loved one's friends, relatives, church members, club members, and business associates to visit, send cards, phone, and send email. Sometimes if people hear the loved one is feeling poorly, they stay away, not knowing if the loved one is really up for visitors. Sometimes, they feel uncomfortable, and they don't know what to do or say. You could be present at the beginning of the visit and help them along until the conversation gets going freely and comfortably.

Let potential visitors know if your loved one isn't up to visitors. If he is in pain, encourage short visits. Encourage people to call before visiting to see if your loved one is up to it. Your loved one may want to schedule visits when he knows his pain medication would be working at maximum.

- If your loved one is quite ill, go through the upcoming TV selections available and make him a suggested list of programs with the channel numbers, days, and times. Sometimes, when one is not feeling well, just going through the extensive list of programming seems like too much of an effort. Often older folks will like watching some of the very old TV shows, from many years ago. This will also help them remember better days of the past.

- Set up the DVR to record some of your loved one's favorite TV shows. If he is sick, sleeping, or visiting with someone when it is on, he will be able to watch it another time. He needs some things to look forward to.

- Purchase some of the inexpensive DVDs of old TV shows and old movies which your loved one enjoys.

- Check out some movie DVDs from your local library which your loved one might enjoy watching. You can also often find used movies for a reasonable price at your local pawn shops or garage sales. Consider purchasing a few of your loved one's favorites. Don't forget to include a few comedies too!

- Take your loved one for a drive through the countryside at any time. Do this often if your loved one enjoys it. Some key times to remember this, if you live in an area that enjoys the four seasons, is in the spring when everything is turning green and leafing out, in the fall to look at the fall colors, and during the holidays to see the Christmas lights. Park along a river or the lake and watch the boat traffic, the fishermen, and the birds.

- See if your loved one wants to plant a few flowers or some vegetable plants.

- Drive to the local root beer stand for a float or ice cream shop for a malted milk.

- Keep your loved one supplied with some good reads, if he's a bookworm. Your local library can keep him reading. Some cities have used bookstores with a good variety of books at a reasonable price. Another option is a book exchange program where individuals can trade books. Maybe your loved one would enjoy getting an electronic reader to use.

Have the Last Laugh on Cancer

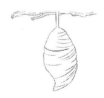

When your loved one received the diagnosis of cancer, life suddenly became very serious. It certainly is a serious illness, but that does not mean that we should take away the joy, benefits, and stress relief of laughter.

One of my most memorable and shocking moments of laughing with or at cancer came to me at a young age. I was in college. It was at a small college with a wonderful faculty who knew their students well. It was a beautiful fall day as our first-period class started. My favorite instructor was teaching the class. He was really getting into his topic and had the class spellbound when we all heard a noise in the back of the room. In the door came one of my classmates. John was a tall, lean, and handsome young man with a wife and child. Mr. Jensen glared at him. We knew he was annoyed that his teaching moment had been interrupted. John didn't appear to be uncomfortable about the situation. He simply said, "I'm sorry I'm late. I was on my way in time, but my leg kept falling off and I had to keep stopping to put it back on." John had lost his leg to cancer and had a prosthetic leg. In that moment, John had put the entire class and the instructor at ease about his cancer. He also helped us laugh, as he did, about what could have been a very discouraging situation.

Bring laughter to your loved one's life! Even if your loved one is going through the fight of his life, he needs something to make him laugh now more than ever. Studies have shown the many psychological benefits of laughter. Laughter can help people cope, heal, and recuperate faster. Laughter is best shared, if possible.

Research has found that one minute of laughter can elevate heart rates to a comparable level of that achieved after ten minutes of exercise. That is amazing! Studies have also indicated that laughter releases endorphins, hormones which are known to cause good feelings. Endorphins reduce stress, assist with sleep, relaxation, and have a positive impact on one's immune system. It has also been shown that laughter increases oxygen use. Laughter has been used to increase pain tolerance. Some doctors have even included fifteen minutes of laughter daily in their recommendations for a healthy lifestyle. Could your loved one use some good feelings and some laughter today?

Here are some ways you can help bring some much-needed laughter into your loved one's life at a time when it would be very beneficial to him:

- Share a funny story.

- There are DVDs created for times like your loved one is going through. Some can be found in department stores. If you do an Internet search, you will find some as well.

- Watch a comedy show on TV or a funny movie.

- Look up some funny videos to watch on the Internet.

- Tell about an embarrassing moment.

- Ask your loved one about some past activity that is funny. He'll probably get a good laugh telling the story again.

- Make a pet do a funny trick.

- Tell about a hilarious comment made by a toddler or preschooler.

- Laugh about funny things that happen throughout the day.

- Perhaps poke some gentle fun at yourself and some of your "issues" or flaws to help your loved one see that he is not the only one with a less-than-perfect body.

Laugh about the disease and issues surrounding it. You may need to help your loved one see how funny some of these issues are and let him initiate the laugh. You certainly don't want him to think you are making light of his disease, but if you can help him see the humor in some of the situations surrounding their disease, it can invoke humor.

You know your loved one. You must decide when it's appropriate to use humor and when not to. Some cancer patients make jokes about their illness, while others don't. The amount and type of humor you use may also depend on just how sick the cancer patient is. This can vary from time to time depending on the current situation. Is the patient currently undergoing chemo? Did they recently have surgery? Are they early in the treatment? What is the prognosis?

The Flagpole Technique

One of the big challenges of caring for a loved one with cancer is trying to keep in touch with how they are feeling on a particular day or at a particular time. It can get tiring if people are continuously asking, "How are you feeling?" You and your loved one could come up with a non-verbal signal to help ease the stress for both of you.

Kim became quite emotional about her health situation. Every day was an effort for her. Soon the strain affected everyone in the family. Previously, she was a very upbeat person. There would be days she could cope, but there were also many very emotional days. At times, it was difficult for family and close friends to know how to talk to her, not knowing what kind of a day she was having.

One day Kim's husband made a little wooden flagpole and stand for her to place in a designated area where most people would easily notice it. Everyone was quite curious. Kim said the flag was to let everyone around her know what kind of a day she was having. If the red flag was displayed, she was having a difficult day. If the red flag was down, it was a good day. Without having to say a word, she was able to help everyone close to her know how to approach her on a particular day.

Would your loved one like to use a signal or keyword to help him communicate his feelings on a particular day without having to discuss it? It could be as simple as your loved one giving you a thumbs-up or thumbs-down signal.

If your loved one is feeling quite ill, he may want you to just sit quietly with him. This might be a time of no talking, just being there. In that case, maybe humor on television would be an option to distract him. Perhaps listening to some of his favorite music would help. Knowing your loved one as you do and learning how the illness is affecting him will help you find the right response.

The Feeding of a Butterfly

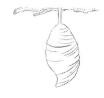

Just as butterflies are picky eaters and only partake of a select diet, so it is with many cancer patients. In fact, did you know that butterflies don't eat? They simply drink nectar.

Ask questions about what your loved one would like to eat.

Eating is often a problem for people with cancer, especially during chemotherapy and as the disease progresses. Often, it helps to stay with simple foods.

Use fresh fruits and vegetables for health and to make the food more appealing. When little else appealed to him, my dad loved fresh strawberries and a special kind of cream of chicken soup. Try to make meals pleasant and appealing. Losing weight is often a concern. Follow the doctor's and nutritionist's recommendations for your loved one's diet. Unless the doctor says to, don't make a big deal out of the quantity of food eaten, to add stress to an already stressful situation. Put a little effort into making the food attractive. Try to think of some pleasant conversation at the table to help keep your loved one's mind off the food; so hopefully, it will be easier for him to force himself to eat a little. Put a small vase of flowers on the table one day. Light a candle another time. Use some china and crystal once in a while. Put on a tablecloth another day. Keep it interesting and appealing.

Work with your loved one's doctor and nutritionist to get some good tips on healthy eating for cancer patients and for those going through chemotherapy and radiation treatments. Nutrition is receiving a lot of attention as an important component of cancer treatment. There are recipe books packed with nutritious recipes specifically for cancer patients. Try a few recipes out on your loved one. If you have some real concerns about your loved one's skimpy diet, talk to the doctor or nurse. They may have some suggestions. They may also have some dietary concerns related to your loved one's treatment. Be sure to pay close attention to those concerns. For some cancer patients, eating can become quite a chore. Anything caregivers can do to make it more pleasant would be a good thing!

Butterfly Finances

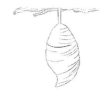

Sometimes you need some financial help. Cancer can take a devastating toll on a family's finances. Most people probably won't know or think about that unless you share that with a trusted friend or family member. They might be the catalyst you need to do something big like a fundraiser or some little things to help take the financial pressure off you and your loved one. Sometimes all you may need is some extra gas money or some extra money for eating out when your loved one is in the hospital.

There are other sources for help as well. Some communities have a local cancer support group that serves as a financial resource to assist local cancer patients and their families. These groups may provide financial assistance to help pay for heating bills in the winter, gas money for doctor visits, or trips for treatments. They also provide volunteers to drive patients to and from treatments. Most people are reluctant to ask for financial help or reduced prices, but sometimes by sharing what the cancer patient is dealing with, help may unexpectedly become available.

Some people have special insurance policies that will provide specific financial benefits for an individual who is cancer-stricken or for their family. For example, there is an insurance company that will pay for a cancer patient's family member to fly home to see them. Perhaps your loved one wants to see his son, but his son doesn't have the cash to purchase an airline ticket. This could help both of them out. Check if your loved one has coverage like this. What a blessing to have such resources available at such a devastating time!

Butterfly Talk

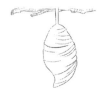

Try to leave the door open to conversation about anything your loved one wants to discuss. Say, "I'm sure there are a lot of things on your mind right now, with what you are dealing with. I'm sure it's not easy to discuss some of them with many people also. For most people, it helps to have someone to talk to and to bounce ideas off of. It helps to have someone to vent to when you are frustrated or upset. I just want you to know that if there's anything that you'd like me to find out for you or that you'd like to talk about, I am available. I can handle whatever it is you want to talk about. You can come to me at any time, so please don't hesitate."

Don't judge. Just listen. If you haven't been in their situation, you really can't understand, but you can empathize that you can only imagine how challenging it must be.

> *Every trip was getting more difficult. As I prepared to leave on the long drive home, I turned back from the door. "I'm dying, you know." My father stated it clearly. He looked deep into my eyes. What could I say? I knew it to be true. "We all are, Dad," I responded softly. "It's just that most of us don't know when." What was Dad's point? He wanted to be sure that I had a reality check. He wanted to see my reaction. After my stepmother told me how my visits made him more upbeat, I had been so focused on trying to maintain that and cheer him up that I hid my feelings of sadness at his prognosis. He wanted me to be prepared.*

It could be that your loved one would feel more comfortable talking about some things with a trusted friend. That may require a phone call to ask them to visit your loved one.

Butterflies are important pollinators. They go from flower to flower slurping the sweet nectar that sustains them. As a by-product, they pollinate those plants. Caregivers pollinate too. You go to family members, friends, and your loved one with cancer, and spread good things, which causes a chain reaction of events to occur. Your interaction with others may cause friends to pay a visit, send a card, make a phone call, or deliver a meal. These are among many things that sustain that feeling of love given to your loved one earlier in the process. All too often, after the initial shock wears off and as the illness progresses, some friends and family don't come around as much as they did previously. They don't want to come out of their comfort zone, especially, if the prognosis is grim. Don't forget to pollinate the area around your loved one by encouraging some of those people to visit or call your loved one.

Butterfly Feelings

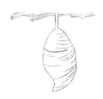

Respect your loved one's wishes to the greatest extent possible. It's his life! Some cancer patients may be at a point where there is little they can control. Honoring your loved one's reasonable wishes are an important thing to help him feel there's still some things he can control. An exception to this would be health and safety issues.

My dad was mentally out of it. His experimental treatment was successfully destroying the cancer, but it was also killing him. My stepmother and I met with the doctor to fill him in on his deteriorating situation. The doctor felt my dad needed to go to a nursing home temporarily until the poison from the experimental drug left his system and he was functioning normally again. Dad was not happy about the situation, but most of the time he was so out of it that he didn't realize where we were going. My stepmother said she'd like to put Dad in the back seat of the car as she drove him to the nursing home. She said that in his altered state of mind, he had been getting into a habit of trying to open the car door as she drove him to appointments. She thought if he sat in the back, my son and I could sit in the back seat with him and monitor him.

As my stepmother drove down the road at fifty-five miles per hour, Dad reached over and grabbed the door handle. He was about to open the door! Fortunately, my stepmother had alerted me to the possibility of this happening so I was watching for this. My son and I intercepted and stopped him. Without a warning, I shudder to think what the outcome would have been.

Encourage your loved one to join a support group. Some areas have local support groups. Another option is to join an online support group. Listening to and speaking to others living with this devastating disease can help calm an anxious patient. Sometimes cancer patients feel uncomfortable discussing some situations with a loved one. Encourage your loved one to visit one-on-one with someone else who has fought the same battle he is fighting.

Give your loved one a journal to keep records about what is going on with his health. With dated entries, he will be able to actively help the doctors with symptoms as related to various aspects of his treatment. This journal can also be a means for your loved one to confide some of his deepest feelings relating to the disease. It can be a form of therapy. If your loved one is unable to keep a journal of his health situation, you may need to. During such an emotional time, it is easy for everyone to get confused about the health specifics regarding when and how long certain things happened. It is also good to document these things by date to help the doctors determine if some of the issues are in conjunction with a change in medications or treatments. If you go to doctor appointments with your loved one, it is very helpful if you have kept a journal or some notes of things you have noticed that may be significant. You can then share your observations with the doctor. As well as helping your loved one's medical team, this may even help you in seeing a pattern and knowing more of what to expect in the days ahead.

Have you ever gotten home from a doctor visit and struggled to remember what he said? You can record the conversations with your loved one's doctor visit. You can share that with family who may have a lot of questions and review it with your loved one. It gets emotional. You may forget something or your loved one may forget something. With the recording available, everyone can be kept accurately informed. By recording the doctor's instructions and comments about the latest test results, you will be leaving the emotion out of it. It is amazing how often more than one person is in the room with the doctor and "hearing" different things from the same conversation. Some doctors may be resistant to your recording the conversation, but assure them you are simply trying to remember everything they say.

Along with you and your loved one's journal entries, there may come a time when you need to monitor your loved one's weight. Writing the weight down along with the date will help keep you both on track with that. Sometimes loved ones forget to weigh themselves or say they have stayed the same weight to avoid worrying family members. At times, some loved ones just get confused with all the emotions that come into play with this disease and really think they haven't lost weight. There are also those loved ones who are simply in denial about the progress of their disease and don't want to acknowledge the weight loss.

The Power of Faith and an Active Spiritual Life

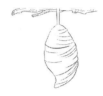

If your loved one has faith, help him with spiritual matters. Keep his clergy informed. Encourage visits from the clergy. Encourage your loved one to go to church, as he feels able to. Make spiritual help available through TV, radio, readings, and devotionals. Because your loved one may have an unpredictable sleep cycle, you may want to set a DVR to record religious broadcasts, so they are available at a time when he feels good enough to watch it. Some religious broadcasts even offer replays of their services over the Internet, available at any time. If your loved one is unable to attend church, you may want to call the clergy to schedule a home visit with your loved one. You can offer to bring in brochures and books to share with your loved one the benefits of having faith during these dark days. If he is feeling poorly, you can offer to read to him. Some religious services are broadcast live on local radio stations.

At certain stages in the cancer process, your loved one may feel anger and possibly even question his faith. Be a sounding board to him at that time to help him work his way through it. If he had faith previously, he will need his faith to help him get through this. Some may have never had a faith before, but may be open to finding out more now. Some people have no interest in the matters of the spirit until they face a devastating illness. Some, at that time, express an interest in learning about spiritual matters. Some are very interested at this time, but don't know how to really express it. They may feel uncomfortable initiating a conversation and not know how to get started. Sometimes, by the caregiver asking him, the conversation will begin.

You can offer to bring in brochures and books. You can suggest TV shows or ask a pastor to visit your loved one to share the benefits of having faith during these dark days.

Perhaps you or a close friend of your loved one could share your faith and ask if your loved one has any specific questions or concerns. You could leave interesting books in the room for your loved one. Sometimes those who put off the matters of faith earlier in their life now face their mortality with fear and regret at not taking care of the matters of faith earlier. This can also be a source of stress for the loved one. Anything you can do to help him with this would be very beneficial to him.

Matters of faith are deeply personal. Some people are very spiritual. Others are not. Some really don't have an interest in spiritual matters until life reminds them of the fact that we are not going to be of this world forever. Some realize they want the assurance of life after death. If you are a person of faith and your loved one is not, this can be very stressful. You cannot force anyone to have faith. It is something that they must want and see a need for. What you can do is to encourage them and set an example for them. You can pray for them and with them. They may not feel they know how to pray. You can explain prayer is speaking to God from the heart. It is a conversation between you and God. You can share your faith with them and offer to have conversations and answer questions. You may not have all the answers. That is when you pray for them and call on the experts to help you out so that your loved one's questions will be answered.

Julie was feeling so stressed. Her father was dying, and she was worried about him spiritually. He never really discussed his beliefs or lack of. He was raised in a family of faith, but he didn't go to church. Julie didn't know where her father was spiritually. She often shared her faith with her father, but he never responded. She struggled with how to talk to him about it. She didn't want to upset him, but she knew if he were to acknowledge and deal with his spiritual life that it would be a great comfort to him now. She considered asking her father if he'd like her to have a pastor visit him.

Before the pastor visit could happen, things progressed quickly with Julie's father's illness. As she was about to talk to him again of matters of faith and the comfort it gives, she realized he was mentally out of it. There was not going to be a chance to have that conversation. Julie was crushed and felt like she had failed her father. As she talked to the hospital chaplain, he gave her comfort when she did not expect any. The chaplain reminded her that we do not know all that happens in those last weeks, days, and minutes with our loved one. The chaplain reminded her that her father may well have come to faith before he slipped away. Those words from the chaplain were a source of comfort to Julie for years to come.

Who are the experts, if you need to call on them, to help your loved one through their spiritual crisis? Hopefully, the expert you call on will already have a relationship with your loved one. If your loved one has a minister, but he has just not been spiritually active, he may or may not be comfortable seeing him. Having a trusted spiritual advisor your loved one already knows and has a relationship with would be preferable.

If your loved one has been in the hospital and gotten to know the hospital chaplain, he may trust him enough to be open to some in-depth spiritual conversations. If your loved one is currently under hospice care, he may have received visits from the hospice chaplain, and established a relationship with him. The hospital and hospice chaplains deal with loved ones and their families in crisis on a regular basis and have a lot of experience in these matters. It is important that you find someone who is used to working with the dying if your loved one is terminal.

Everyone has different gifts. Some pastors and family ministers have a wonderful gift of being good listeners and are able to get the cancer patient to open up with their concerns. If the loved one with cancer does not have an existing relationship with the clergy or a family minister, perhaps they are starting to build one with a hospital chaplain, hospice chaplain, or counselor with experience helping the dying. If not, you might suggest they start seeing one of them, so they can start to build that relationship. You will need to ask him who he would like to see and help make arrangements for the visit. Make it as easy as you can to help your loved one with this.

They need that relationship to ensure trust. Without the trust factor, it will be difficult for your loved one to be open and honest enough to reveal his deepest and most heartfelt concerns. In other words, this is a process that cannot be rushed. It is going to take time and patience for your loved one to become comfortable with someone new. It will take time for him to learn to trust and open up to someone new.

It is important to address the need for resolving your loved one's spiritual needs and concerns early in the process. Some cancers are diagnosed late. Some cancers progress rapidly. You will not know the extent of the cancer right away. You will not know how much time you have available to lovingly help your loved one address these important matters. Sometimes a loved one can quickly become mentally out of it, or go into a coma. Do not underestimate the importance of spiritual care. At first much of the focus is put on medical matters, but do not wait too long to address spiritual matters. It can mean all the difference in whether or not your loved one and his family have peace. It is important to help your loved one find peace at this difficult time.

Healing Broken Relationships

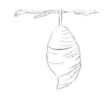

You may know of some long-harbored resentment between your loved one and an old friend or a family member, or perhaps even yourself. It is very healing for people to mend old wounds and correct past mistakes. This is especially true if your loved one is in a terminal situation. Some people near the end of their lives see the error of their ways. Many want to correct these past transgressions regardless of who was wrong before they pass away. This is a delicate situation, but you may be able to help them. Be an ambassador for the healing process of forgiveness, if it serves your loved one well.

It's not easy for everyone to show their love to others. Through this illness, some people learn to do so, while others continue to struggle with it. You may be able to help your loved one show his love to someone who desperately needs to feel their love at such a time. You may also be able to help another who has never expressed their love for your loved one with cancer to show their love. You will often need to be the encourager for all who are uncomfortable dealing with these feelings and the toll the illness has taken on your loved one. Perhaps you could help initiate such a conversation. Sometimes pastors or family ministers are helpful in initiating these kinds of conversations. If you are very fortunate, you may have the services of an oncology chaplain who can help you work through this. Hospital social workers are another option available to you at times.

More clinics are designing an oncology team with trained staff to help you and your loved one deal with the entire scope of the illness and its impact on you and your loved one's life. Sometimes hospital or hospice chaplains can help facilitate dealing with some of these issues. Remember, this can be a very emotional time for your loved one. Some are unable to have these kinds of conversations, but may feel troubled. If your loved one is unable to discuss these matters, he may find it easier to just write a letter to the person he wishes to create a better connection with. Later, perhaps they can meet and have a conversation. This is often a time of life when loved ones have regrets and feel the need to make things right. Priorities in life tend to come into focus more clearly when facing a devastating illness. When your loved one addresses these situations, it helps relieve stress and helps him find peace.

The Power of Touch

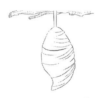

As a caregiver, you should use the power of touch. Touch your loved one. The power of touch is universal.

Massage therapy is used for some cancer patients. A specifically trained massage therapist will consider the patient's particular type of cancer as a plan is devised. Sometimes massage therapy can also be used during end-of-life, and as a method of relaxation for cancer survivors and for cancer caregivers. Although the touch of a massage therapist is of great value, the touch of a loved one or a friend will mean more because of the social connection.

Encouraging news came out of a recent study of family caregivers receiving a minimal amount of training on touching techniques. It was determined that caregivers can provide their loved ones benefits nearly as effectively as professionals. The study revealed that the most beneficial impact was that of a reduction in stress and anxiety, followed by a positive impact on pain, fatigue, depression, and nausea.

Give your loved one a generous amount of hugs, but be gentle if they are hurting. Yes, you can sometimes forget to be careful and cause your frail loved one some unintentional pain. It's good to ask if they are having pain before you hug or massage them.

Speak the language of touch. Physical touching says so much. Touch speaks loudly; touch speaks softly. Touch is gentle. Touch is endearing. Touch is a language all its own. Touch speaks of love. Touch says you care. Hold their hand. Gently touch their shoulder. Stroke their hair.

Emotional Touch

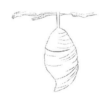

We know that physical touching has a strong impact on people. Another powerful form of touch is emotional touch. Make eye contact with your loved one. Look into his eyes and see inside his heart. Sometimes this hurts you, but it is important. Many people feel so sad and uncomfortable about your loved one's illness that they avoid eye contact. Your loved one sees and feels that. He needs those who are close to him to connect with him.

Tell your loved one that you love him. Don't go about thinking he knows that you love him. You may show it, but that's not enough. Actually say it again. He needs to hear that now more than ever. This may be a cause of discomfort for some people. Some grow up in homes where little affection is displayed and even less verbal acknowledgement of affection is demonstrated. Others grow up in homes that are very verbal and affectionate. Some of us grew up in homes where even the visiting boyfriends got kissed goodnight by the siblings! The point is, your loved one needs to hear that you love them. He may feel he is a burden to you. He may wonder if he still is thought of as someone of worth, simply because of his illness and inability to contribute as he did in the past. Reassure him that the love is still there.

Reminisce about happy memories in the presence of your loved one. Those happy memories will trigger an emotional response. They will often bring a sense of calm to your loved one.

Mom was in a coma-like state. Her breathing was very erratic. She was having sporadic episodes of defibrillation. We were sure she would not come out of it. One evening, all seven of her children sat around her bedside. We knew the end was near. No one spoke it, but that truth was in the air. As mother's erratic breathing continued, we started speaking of old times. That entire evening, we reminisced about funny childhood events. We hashed over fond memories of growing up together. With seven children there were lots of interesting stories to tell. We spoke of childhood mischief, holidays, and many happier times. The later it got, one-by-one some of her children nodded off to sleep in the hard hospital chairs. Those who were still awake continued reminiscing. Mother's breathing soon became slow and steady. I really believe she heard our conversations about all the good old days. I truly believe hearing her children rehash fond memories was a comfort to her at that time. I also believe it was a comfort to her to know that her children had so many fond memories of their childhood, which she played such a large role in.

During those last hours, my stepdad sat by her side and accepted what was happening. In a final act of love, he gave her his permission to leave. He picked up her hand, leaned over by her ear, and said, "It's okay to go. Go to God." That was the best gift he could give her at that time. We all cried. In a matter of a few hours—she did just that—she went to God. He had given her permission to go. She could now stop struggling and break free of her cocoon of love. She was free to fly to God. After being in a coma for several days, she opened her white, glazed eyes. She looked towards the door. Her eyes followed from the door all the way to the window on the opposite side of the room. It was as if she saw something or someone come in the door and exit through the window of her room. She closed her eyes again and took her last breath. My stepdad gave her a gift. She, in turn, gave him and her children a gift.

So many of the little things you do with your loved one provide an emotional touch. Listen to him. It shows you care. Sit with him. Sit with him in silence, if that's what he wants. Ask if there's anything he would like to talk about. Encourage him to feel free to talk. You are there to listen without judgment.

Sometimes you need to emotionally touch your loved one. You need to learn how to create a feeling of love during a time when so many stressors are entering your loved one's life. It's the little things that mean a lot right now. The little loving thoughts and deeds help you to be in tune with your loved one. Do it all with love. It won't be without challenges and heartache. That's all part of the process. No one said the journey would be easy. You must learn to look beyond your feelings. You must learn to look beyond the cocoon.

Love manifests itself in many ways. For the cancer victim, many expressions you would consider insignificant, are touching examples of love. Your loved one may not express it, but the acts of love you do encase and permeate your loved one's cocoon. It incubates within and helps create a beautiful thing.

~ Susan Brownell ~

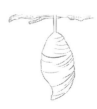

The emotional touch of caregiving
leaves a fingerprint on your loved one's heart.

~ Susan Brownell ~

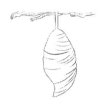

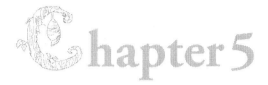

Chapter 5

Cocoon Care for You: Surround Yourself with Love for Self-Care

Learn to get in touch with the silence within yourself,
and know that everything in life has purpose.
There are no mistakes, no coincidences,
All events are blessings given to us to learn from.

~ Elisabeth-Kubler-Ross ~

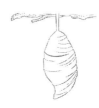

Be on your guard; stand firm in the faith;
be men of courage be strong.

~ 1 Corinthians 16:13 ~

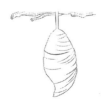

The ultimate lesson all of us have to learn is unconditional love, which includes not only others, but ourselves as well.

~ Elisabeth-Kubler-Ross ~

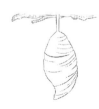

One of the first questions most caregivers ask themselves is, "Why?" Why is my loved one afflicted with this terrible disease? Why must my loved one suffer and possibly even die? Why must our lives be so disrupted by this devastating illness? Why must my loved one suffer the effects of the treatments? Why do I have to endure the daunting task of caring for my loved one when it hurts me so badly?

It's important to assess these thoughts as early as you can. Find a quiet place where you can have some alone time. You need some time to think deeply. Focus on what is happening with your loved one. Think about the implications for his life, your life, and the lives of all who care for your loved one. Even though you may not know what the reason is, tell yourself there is a reason for this. Be ready to receive the reason when and if it is unveiled.

Try to find some quiet time alone on a regular basis. Even if it's not for long blocks of time, it can be rejuvenating. Think of this as something important you can do for your mental health. It is good to have some quiet time to think. Many things are happening in your life right now. You need a little uninterrupted quiet time to assess what is happening.

What good could possibly come from this situation? How can anyone call an event like cancer a blessing? What life lesson is being taught? Who is the learner in that life lesson? Perhaps there's more than one learner in this life lesson.

If you've never been one to pay attention to life events and analyze their impact, now is the time to start. Think about what you know about yourself and your loved one as you enter the caregiver process. Revisit this often in the coming days, weeks, and months. Journaling can help you with this process. Compare your observations over time. You will be astonished at how much you learn about yourself and your loved one. You may also be amazed to discover some hidden blessings scattered throughout the experience.

You may become closer to your loved one. You may become a stronger, better person for the experience. You may improve your relationships as a result of this experience. You may even change your life's priorities.

Be open and ready to receive the great lessons about to be unveiled. You must pay attention, but the lessons will reveal themselves one by one. Some of those life lessons may not come to light until long after the battle with cancer is over. Acknowledge those lessons and the impact on your life as they occur.

Do you know any people who are constantly busy and involved in just about anything and everything? How do they do it? Do they ever get tired? Do they have any limits at all? Do they get enough sleep and family time? Do they take time to sit down and enjoy a good, nutritious meal? We all have our various priorities. We all have different levels of tolerance. We all have different levels of health and fitness.

I took care of my family. I visited my dad and tried to help from a distance. I only missed a couple of days of work during Dad's long illness. I helped plan my daughter's wedding. I made bouquets and floral centerpieces for her wedding. I really don't know how I did it all. Besides working full-time, I was teaching out of town part-time two nights a week. I had a lot of homework papers to correct in the evenings.

I wasn't getting enough sleep and was stressed about Dad's illness, keeping up with both jobs, and driving the 130 miles each way every time I went to see him. I was getting tired. I remembered what my stepmother said about how my visits perked him up. I knew I had to just keep going. Somehow I had to dig into my innermost being and just keep going.

It had become obvious that the end was getting near for Dad, and I felt I needed to go as often as I could. I was planning to go visit Dad on Saturday. I was feeling stressed at what kind of condition I would find him in when I got there. Suddenly, I wasn't feeling so good. My fibromyalgia got so out of control that I ended up sick in bed with a severe headache, vomiting, and severe pain. I could barely turn my neck. I was so sick I couldn't drive the two and a half hours to go see Dad the last two weeks of his life.

I had failed to take care of myself when my dad was sick and dying. I had such guilt that I was unable to be there for him and my stepmother at that time. In going overboard, I was trying to be a superwoman and be all things for all people. I had over-extended myself. Yes, I had neglected myself. In an effort to do as much as I could for everyone except myself, I failed to be there when it mattered most. In my effort to be and do all I could to surround my Dad with my love, I had messed up, and I felt horrible. I felt like I had failed him and failed my stepmother when they both needed me most. Guilt overcame me.

You're doing a great job taking care of your loved one! Now it's time to take care of yourself and your family. It's time for some Cocoon Care for you. Surround yourself with love. Start by loving yourself and showing it. How do you show it? You take some time for rest and relaxation. You take the time to prepare or buy a nutritious meal. You somehow find time to get some exercise. You get enough sleep. How? You need to get creative.

Caregivers are givers. As givers, they can get pretty busy and often tend to neglect themselves. This can be very serious. Caregivers are often under a tremendous amount of stress. Caregivers can experience a high rate of burnout. If caregivers neglect themselves as they deal with all the work and stress of caregiving to a loved one with cancer, they are setting themselves up for health problems and depression. You must keep your priorities in order to stay healthy. You need your health now, more than ever. Your loved one needs you healthy too.

The solution is to remember to place caring for yourself as one of your top priorities. This is not easy to do. It takes discipline. But, it can be done.

So, how do you do it? Can you feel the love? Ideally, you should surround yourself with love. All of that love doesn't have to come from others.

Understanding Your Loved One and Yourself

Caring for a loved one with cancer is an emotional challenge. If that loved one is a spouse, it can be especially difficult and can put a strain on a marriage. The cancer journey can also act as a bond, bringing a loved one and spouse even closer together. Caring for a parent or child with cancer can also be emotionally draining and stressful as roles change.

Not every cancer patient responds the same. Not every caregiver to a loved one with cancer responds the same either. Both you and your loved one are dealing with a lot of uncertainty. Sometimes a loved one will push the ones he loves the most away. He may be having a hard time dealing with what comes next on this journey. He may respond with feelings of being smothered. He may feel you and the rest of the family are being overly protective and express a need for some space. He may have the perception that he is seen as broken, someone to be pitied, and even worse, worthless. He may feel he is a burden to his family and be stressed by that. He, as well as you, the caregiver, may suffer from emotional exhaustion.

There may be times when you feel like you don't even know your loved one. He may say something hurtful to you or a family member. Some cancer patients, who used to always be nice to be around, can suddenly become very difficult and agitated. Sometimes those individuals who were always a challenge to live with may become extremely difficult to live with after receiving a cancer diagnosis. Remember, you may be seeing changes due to your loved one's current medical situation or as a result of the drugs he has been administered. Communicate your concerns to your loved one's medical team about major changes you have observed in your loved one. They may be able to help. Some cancer patients become so depressed they must be prescribed anti-depressants.

Other cancer patients will serve as a source of inspiration to those around them as they handle their devastating illness with grace and dignity. Some cancer patients will feel ill a lot, while others not so much. Some will have a lot of pain, while others not so much.

During this process there may be times that you both must deal with sadness, insomnia, loneliness, worry, fear, and a host of other emotions.

If you feel you aren't handling these emotions very well after you have had some time to adjust, consider joining a support group for caregivers. Support groups can be very beneficial as you learn what you are feeling is not all that uncommon. You will learn how others have gotten through difficult times. You will encounter many understanding, non-judgmental, and supportive individuals in these groups. Some of these groups meet locally face-to-face, or you can do some online searches to find support groups available online twenty-four hours a day. If you are house-bound because your loved one is terminal, the online support groups will be easier to access and a source of continuity as your loved one declines.

It is very important for you to recognize that the feelings of anger, sadness, and even some resentment are all normal responses to your situations. Sometimes it is all right to not be okay with the situation you find yourself in. That is a normal response. Sometimes you may even have to feel a bit sorry for yourself. The important thing is to not get permanently stuck in this mindset. If you must have a brief pity party, go ahead and indulge yourself, then move on to something positive and constructive. You are only given so much energy to expend. Use it wisely.

Acceptance can be a difficult place for caregivers and cancer patients to arrive at. If your loved one is diagnosed as terminal, many doctors don't want to take a patient's hope away. Hope is very powerful. Miracles can and do happen. Unfortunately, they don't happen every time we would like one. Sometimes, it becomes necessary to accept the inevitable. That can be very difficult. Sometimes decisions need to be made and wishes need to be honored. Sometimes for one's own mental well-being, acceptance of reality must occur. Although it may be difficult, it can also be freeing to reach a point of acceptance.

We live in an information age. At times that is wonderful. We can find information quickly and easily. We know what is happening all over the globe. We hear the good news of the day, and we hear the upsetting news of the day. Sometimes, we feel it is too much. Too much information. Too much stress. Too much contact. There's so much happening all around us, yet to the cancer caregiver and the loved one with cancer, the world is a smaller place. Their world revolves around dealing with a devastating illness. Most of their emotions are spent on dealing with what is happening in their small world. They do not have the time or the energy to deal with much of the rest.

How to Surround Yourself with Love

Allow yourself to feel self-love. Respect yourself for the generous act of caregiving which you are doing. Give yourself credit. Love yourself for who you are. Eliminate your self-criticism. If you think you aren't doing anything important, make a list of your positive qualities. List what you have done for your loved one today, this week, and this month. Your list is probably longer than you expected.

Mindset

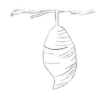

One of the most important things for a caregiver is having a good mindset. This is essential to providing care while still taking care of yourself. You need to try to remain positive. This is not always easy if your loved one is seriously ill. It's not easy if you are feeling exhausted or stressed. How do you get and maintain a good outlook on such a situation?

Use positive affirmations. Affirmations are statements you read or recite to yourself daily to bring about positive thinking and self-empowerment.

Use positive self-talk. As things happen and you mentally react, avoid negative responses. Tell yourself you can do it. Envision yourself being a capable, successful caregiver. Visualize yourself asking others for help when you need it.

Don't be too hard on yourself. For example, tell yourself, "Pace yourself. It's only Monday. You don't have to do it all in one day."

Are you new to caring for a loved one with cancer? Are you scared and overwhelmed? Mindset is so important to your ability to cope. Do what you must to get in the right mindset to give care. When feeling overwhelmed, remember the old childhood story. "I think I can. I think I can!" I like to add one more statement to that: "I know I can!" One good way to overcome the feeling of being overwhelmed is to make a list of the tasks and responsibilities and identify what you need to do now, in the near future, and in the distant future.

Keep things in perspective. Instead of telling yourself you shouldn't take time to get some extra sleep or watch your favorite TV show, remind yourself doing some of those things are actually good for you! It is not a "treat" to get eight hours of sleep at night. It is a requirement of your body to keep it performing well. It is not necessarily a "treat" to take an hour and watch your favorite TV show. It is one of many ways you can exercise your right and need to give yourself some emotional release from your challenging new reality. It is a small thing you can do for your mental health and wellbeing.

Keep things positive. You are under enough stress. Stay away from all things negative, including negative people. They will only drag you down. You do not have the energy to deal with them.

Recognize that it is perfectly normal to feel a sense of loss, anger, and yes, even sometimes resentment for what this disease has done to your loved one, yourself, and your family. You may feel it is not fair. Cancer never is fair. You may feel you and your loved one have been or will be robbed of precious time together. That is a normal response. Acknowledge it, accept it, and then move on to dealing with the situation at hand.

Avoid the negative media to help promote a positive mindset. There is so much negativity in the world today. If listening to the doom and gloom newscasts gets you down, don't watch them. If there's something really big going on that you need to know about, chances are that you'll hear about it from someone.

Don't let little things get to you at work or in relationships. This can drain you of energy you need to do constructive things. Recognize you have only a specific amount of energy. Prioritize what you will let consume that energy. Guard that energy as if it were money in your wallet.

Focus on what's important. Recognize that you can't do it all. Recognize that you can't control everything that's going on. That's okay. What if the caterpillar got worried about the robin having difficulty pulling that worm out of the hard, dry soil in the back yard? What if the concerned caterpillar worried if his friends would break out of their cocoons before him and beat him to the flowers with the best nectar? What if the caterpillar stressed over which twig to attach itself to because of the possibility of a potential storm causing a branch to break off the tree? If the caterpillar got so wrapped up in all the little things going on around it, would it ever get its cocoon completed?

Reading, TV, Movies

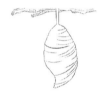

With all the things you have to do, is there really time for TV? Yes, if you choose to make it so.

Take time for your favorite TV show. Set your DVR to record every episode if you have to. Depending on how much care your loved one requires, it is possible that your loved one may interrupt the viewing of your favorite show. You will also have times that you will receive a lot of phone calls from concerned friends, relatives, and co-workers. Rather than get upset or resentful about these interruptions, plan for them, so you have access to watch your favorite show later, if necessary. If time is an issue when trying to watch it, use the skip feature on your remote to get through commercials and dull areas, so you can get the gist of it. You need to hang on to some things that are special to you so you have some things to look forward to.

Watch a favorite movie that you know will make you feel good. Some like to focus on comedies, "chick flicks", and old favorite movies. Science fiction movies are good to get lost in and can help you temporarily forget about everything else. Once or twice a week try to find time to look at the upcoming broadcast schedule and set your DVR to record these favorites so you don't have to be concerned about interruptions.

Lose yourself in a TV series or soap opera. This gives you something to talk to others about during those times you aren't getting out much.

Record a favorite old or current comedy show. Watch one every night to help you laugh, relax, and unwind. Comedy can really help get you through some of the rough spots.

Read a favorite book or magazine. What's on the best-seller list? Is there something captivating that you can look forward to continuing from day to day?

Get inspired! Get yourself an inspirational calendar or an inspirational book with daily readings to uplift and encourage you. Get in the habit of reading this every morning or every night. Short readings easily fit into a busy schedule and can set the tone for a good day.

Exercise

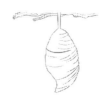

Unless you have been strictly following an exercise schedule before you go into the caregiver mode, you may feel quite tempted to eliminate or greatly reduce the amount of exercise you do. With the number of doctor appointments, treatments, and the complete upheaval of any kind of a normal schedule, it may seem very difficult to work exercise into your schedule. Don't succumb to the temptation!

For all those who like to give reasons why they can't, don't want to, or shouldn't exercise, take note of the following information which will help you convince yourself of the value of exercise. Exercise is an antidote to stress!

Why you need to maintain an exercise schedule

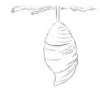

Regular exercise will help you with stress management. It's just too easy to put off exercising. Most of us don't like it. It's one of many ways you can take care of yourself—the caregiver! Simply put, exercise makes you feel better.

After you start reaping the rewards of exercise, you may be surprised to find you actually start looking forward to it. Exercise increases your endorphins. It's that "feel good" feeling you get after exercising. Exercise helps lessen depression, a common problem with caregivers.

As you work out, you will probably feel the tension begin to leave your body. Caregivers often carry a lot of tension. You may not even be aware of it after it has become a habit. Clenching the jaw, tensing the muscles in your arm or leg, and getting a stiff neck or shoulders can all be indicators of tension.

Exercise gives you time to self-reflect. This is time that is hard to come by as a caregiver. You are actually accomplishing two things at once by exercising and giving yourself some quiet time to think. As strange as it may seem, sometimes as a caregiver, there isn't even time to just sit and think and reflect on what is happening. It's very difficult to deal with a situation when you don't even have time to think about it.

Exercise can allow you to multi-task. You know that favorite TV show you recorded, but didn't feel you had time to watch? Given the right circumstances, you may be able to watch it while you exercise. If you use a treadmill at your house, or some other piece of exercise equipment, you can play the recorded show on a TV in front of your workout equipment. Do you have an audio book you've been looking for the time to listen to? Do that when you exercise.

For many, exercise provides a burst of energy. Your mood improves with exercise. What caregiver couldn't use an improved mood?

Exercise can also be a social event. If you go to the gym or walk with a friend, that can reap you the additional rewards of face-to-face contact with another. Life can easily become somewhat isolated when you are a caregiver. You need to try to maintain some social connections.

What exercise will do for you

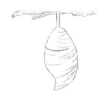

Exercise will help you feel better mentally and physically. Exercise will help you with weight control. As caregivers get bogged down in their daily tasks, they struggle to maintain an exercise program. Caregivers spend considerable time at hospitals and clinics and may not always have access to good meals. As a result, some extra pounds might start to creep on.

Think of all the health problems that can be avoided or minimized by exercise. Exercise is also good for relieving stress.

How you can make it doable

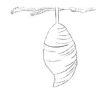

If your loved one is in the hospital:

- Walk up and down several flights of stairs.

- Walk up and down the hallways repeatedly.

- Walk in place in front of the visitors room TV.

- Do stretching exercises in the visitor's room or your loved one's room.

- Use a chair to do exercises. Do leg lifts.

Use a stretching DVD at home. Use a dance or workout DVD at home. Listen to some of your favorite music with the right beat and gait.

Plan your schedule ahead of time. If there's no pattern to your daily activities that will allow a regular schedule, make appointments with yourself on your calendar to fit around your schedule of events. Make it a social event. If you can, involve a friend or the entire family.

Set a reasonable goal for the amount of time and number of days a week you will exercise. Make yourself a chart or checklist to monitor yourself. Realize you may need some flexibility. If your loved one's situation changes, you may need to discontinue your normal exercise activity for a while and improvise. Be flexible...in your mindset! Don't stress out if you have an interruption to your normal routine. Make it your goal to adapt and overcome.

Try various types of exercise until you find what you enjoy. If you enjoy it, you will be more likely to be motivated to continue it. If all else fails, simply take a walk. Walking is excellent exercise.

Remind yourself that you don't have to have bulging biceps to reap the benefits of exercise. You don't have to be the fitness person of the month at the local workout club. Just be yourself and take care of yourself!

Remember to consult with your doctor if you haven't been exercising and you are thinking of beginning an exercise program. Research safe practices to avoid injury. Have something on hand so you can ice yourself in case of injury.

Diet

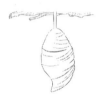

Keeping a healthy, nutritious diet can suddenly become a challenge when faced with the extra demands of caregiving. Keep a good supply of items in your freezer, such as high-quality frozen dinners. Make sure you purchase the kinds with minimal processing, if possible. Focus on dinners that contain a respectable amount of protein and vegetables. Keep some bags of frozen veggies on hand to supplement the frozen dinners. They seldom have enough veggies. If you have trouble getting to the store often enough to keep fresh produce on hand, keep some frozen or canned fruit on hand also for those times when you are out of fresh fruit. Make a menu list of some of you and your loved one's favorite meals, so when you simply can't think of anything, you can look at this list.

Fresh fruits can be appealing and appetizing when little else is. When time allows, make homemade soup. It is much more appealing than the canned. By making a large batch of soup, you can freeze some ahead for future meals. You can also load it up with nutrient-rich vegetables, by cooking the vegetables in the soup broth.

If you want some quick and easy meals from scratch, try some of these:

1. Grill frozen chicken breast pieces. Stir fry some frozen vegetables in olive oil.

2. Bake thawed salmon pieces and top them with apricot preserves the last five minutes. Put some potatoes in the oven to bake and add a veggie.

3. Wrap several potatoes in aluminum foil and place in the oven to bake. Bake pork chops for an hour in the oven. Make some quick and easy baked beans (made from canned pork & beans with a little ketchup and a small amount of brown sugar and a couple of slices of fried bacon). It is even possible to bake raw, peeled mini carrots in their own juice with a little butter and brown sugar.

4. Salad meals are also easy. Prepare lettuce, tomatoes, onions, radishes, cucumbers, and any other salad toppings you like. Fry frozen chicken breast pieces and place the warm chicken on the lettuce salad. Top with your favorite dressing. If you had some leftover chicken you could put cold chicken on it. You can also pick up a roasted chicken from any deli to use on the salad. Sprinkle a few cashews or some sunflower seeds on top for a real treat.

Keep some ginger ale and saltines on hand for when you or your loved one have an upset stomach. Make sure it is real ginger ale. Some do not contain real ginger and don't help with settling your stomach. Another option is to have some ginger cookies on hand. Of course, it never hurts to have a few cans of chicken noodle soup on hand either for those times when either of you have an upset stomach.

Keep in mind that medicines your loved one takes as part of his treatment can affect his taste. Things that used to be favorites can suddenly not taste good anymore. It has nothing to do with your cooking!

When time allows, cook some good homemade meals. There are several good cookbooks available specifically for cancer patients. You may find that you like the food in those too! They have recipes formulated to be appealing to those who are undergoing cancer treatment. You will find these in large bookstores or online. Some are written by family members who have struggled with creating recipes their loved ones would eat. Having a sense of what to cook, related to time management and appeal, will help relieve some stress. Often oven meals or slow cooker meals are user-friendly, but they do require some prior planning. It can be challenging to get cancer patients to eat as they should. It can also be challenging to cook healthy meals when juggling caregiving and trips to the doctor.

What About Your Doctor Visit?

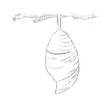

Don't put off taking care of YOU. If it's time for your routine checkup, go do it. If you normally get a flu shot, be sure to keep up with that. You will be under more stress than usual, which will lower your resistance to fighting infections.

Keep a supply of general pharmacy items on hand, so if needed, you don't have to make a special trip to the store. Purchase aspirin, cold remedies, antihistamines, nasal sprays, and other items you use if you have the common cold or flu. It might be helpful to keep some face masks on hand to protect your loved one when you are ill.

If you become ill while caring for your loved one, seek treatment. You don't want to expose your loved one unnecessarily. If you think you have a sinus infection, go to the doctor to get the antibiotics you need to get rid of it. Be sure you tell your doctor you are a caregiver and the kind of contact and proximity you have to your loved one. This may make a difference in how he treats you. For example, some cancer patients undergoing treatments have to be extremely careful to avoid infections. You won't be any help to your loved one if you are sick and unable to help give care to him. If you have trouble getting away to seek treatment, ask a friend or neighbor to sit with your loved one after work. Many health care facilities have an after-hours urgent care clinic available on a walk-in basis. Just be sure to go early enough so you have time to pick up any prescriptions you may need before the pharmacies close.

You may be afraid to go to the doctor. You may be worried you have a serious illness. Do not put off going to the doctor. Sometimes people worry needlessly about symptoms that aren't all that serious. Sometimes the stress of caregiving can make people sick. You won't know what is going on for sure until you are seen by a physician, so go take care of it. The sooner you address the problem, the sooner you can treat it and get well. You owe this to yourself and your loved one.

Learn When to Set Limits

One of the most difficult things caregivers have to learn is when to draw the line between complete devotion to their ill loved one and the stability of their own health. When the caregiver is dealing with an infringement on his or her own health and well-being, it is time to reassess the caregiving situation.

As discussed previously, not everyone with cancer responds the same to this life event. The same can be said for caregivers. Personalities, health situations, the amount of friend and family support, the staging of the disease, the prognosis, and a host of other variables all have an effect on how both the loved one and the caregiver respond, react, and interact with each other.

Unfortunately, some loved ones with cancer can be very challenging, and at times even difficult to deal with. Some have been known to get mean, ornery, and lash out at their loved ones in hurtful ways. Some put their caregivers through unending demands as well as verbal abuse to the caregiver and the loved one's family.

Be compassionate. Be understanding—with your loved one and yourself. The closer your relationship, the more likely you will experience some of their anger and resentment. It's sad, but true. Don't take it personally. Sometimes it isn't the loved one talking. Sometimes it is the illness or the side effects of the treatments or medications causing outbursts of anger and hurtful comments. Remember, your loved one may even look okay, but may be feeling miserable. Sometimes a loved one may try to put on an act for their family to "spare" the family from feeling bad for them. If your loved one just sits in his chair and doesn't DO anything, consider it could be that he just plain doesn't feel good!

When situations get so out of control, you may need to have a break. You may also need to have a heart-to-heart talk with your loved one, if you feel he would understand what you are telling him.

Sometimes, you may have to say no. When the situation gets to the point of severely impacting you and your health, you have to set limits. You may have to call on other family or friends for assistance. You may have to arrange for a respite care break for your loved one to protect your own well-being. You may have to get your loved one's doctor, nurse, or your loved one's hospice team involved to assist you. It can be very difficult to set limits and say no. This can cause caregivers to feel inadequate, guilty, and ashamed. The caregiver may worry, "What will others think?" If the caregiver has no support system, this can be extremely challenging. Do not give up! Keep looking for resources and asking for help. Your health and well-being depends on it.

Relax

Different things help people relax. What might be relaxing for one person might actually be a source of stress or irritation for another. Pay attention to what really feels calming and relaxing to you. Once you know what that is, do it as often as possible.

Perhaps you will want to light a scented candle. Maybe if you turn the lights down low you would find that soothing. Take a relaxing bath. Take a walk on a nature trail. Lather up with one of your favorite scented body creams. Drink a warm cup of tea. Put your feet up. Find that special thing that helps take you to another, more peaceful place and practice that as often as you can.

There are many possibilities for relaxation. The challenge lies in remembering them when you need them and actually taking the time to implement them. You may find you need to leave yourself a reminder. Place a sticky note on the bathroom mirror or the refrigerator saying, "Did you _____ today?" until you have gotten into the habit.

Music

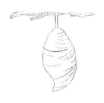

Music has a wonderful ability to soothe—if it's the right kind. For many people, piano music is soothing. For others, acoustic guitar music is very relaxing. Since everyone has their own tastes, this becomes an individual matter. Whatever your favorite and most soothing music is, you should be using it to help you relax. When you are especially stressed, this is one of many things for you to try.

There are many beautiful and relaxing CDs with piano music and acoustic guitars. Harp music is often used as music therapy in nursing homes. For those who enjoy harp music, look for options to purchase harp music CDs. Having some relaxing music playing in the background can be very soothing. Some people like to have a CD playing some relaxing music when they have difficulty sleeping. It can help you relax, sleep, and provide some serenity.

Nature

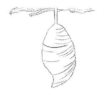

Perhaps one of the best sources of relaxation is enjoying nature and the great outdoors. When you are overwhelmed it is hard to think of even simple, everyday options available. Here's a list of simple, inexpensive, easy-access things that you might find enjoyable and relaxing:

- Plant and work in a vegetable garden.

- Plant and care for flowers outside. When time is a concern, you can quickly and easily plant pots of flowers outside. If you plant them in potting soil, they require virtually no weeding and are quick to water and care for.

- Go on a nature walk.

- Go to the park.

- Watch the birds.

- Feed the ducks at the park.

- Sit on a park bench by a river or lake and watch the water.

- Go to the zoo.

- Visit a botanical garden.

- Visit a butterfly garden.

- Watch a TV documentary with a nature theme.

- Take a short drive on a country road.

- Go to the summer series "Concert in the Park".

- When winter looms over you, visit websites with pictures and videos of warmer, sunnier places.

- Set up a digital picture frame for yourself. Just as they can help your loved one, they can also help you. Load this one with images that make you feel peaceful, happy, loved. Load it with happy images of good times past. Include things you always want to remember. Load up family and friend pictures and vacation and holiday pictures. Insert a lot of nature pictures. Take photos of flowers, snow, lakes, rivers, parks, wild animals, and birds. You can even purchase images or get free images of nature on the Internet. Include pictures of pets, too, for that feel-good feeling. When you are feeling stressed, sit down a few minutes, put your feet up, and lose yourself in these peaceful, happy images.

Sleep

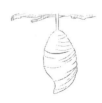

Sleep is an important item. All too often, caregivers faced with too much to do and too little time tend to skimp on sleep. It is important to remember as you retire for the night that you try to shut down your mind's continuous chatter. This may take a little extra effort to accomplish. Here are some suggestions:

- Get a sleep-inducing CD.

- Get regular and sufficient amounts of sleep.

- Try to go to bed and get up around the same time each day so you feel your best. This will also help keep you from being tempted to overdo.

- If you have trouble falling asleep, try this: Get completely ready for bed a half hour to an hour before bedtime. Brush your teeth, wash your face, and put your pajamas on. Now sit and watch a half hour to an hour of TV, or read a book, or listen to some soothing music. Since you are completely ready for bed, you can relax until you are ready to retire for the night. Sometimes having to get ready for bed right at bedtime can wake people up and cause them to be more alert.

People in Your Life: Friends, Relationships & Support

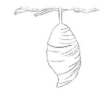

With all the things going on in your life, it would be easy to neglect your friends and extended family. They can do much to help encourage and assist you.

Don't get so wrapped up in all of this that you cut yourself off from family and friends. You really need them right now. How can you most easily maintain contact?

- Phone a friend.

- Visit a friend.

- Email a friend or send a mass email updating friends and family.

- Use social media, when you need to give a quick update to friends, if it's not too personal.

- Lean on your friends and family as you need to. You don't need to do this alone! If you can find a source of support and encouragement in your inner circle, you'll want to tap into this.

- Seek volunteers to help with the work, errands, and appointments. Consider getting help from friends, family, Faith-in-Action, and other community and religious groups.

- Love and appreciate everyone in your life. Look for the good in others. Value all persons and lives as sacred. Be thankful for all who are not ill.

Work

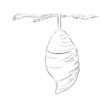

When you are feeling exhausted as you try to work and give care, remind yourself of what you have to be grateful for. Perhaps your loved one can't work right now because he is so sick. Be thankful that you are still able to enjoy working and be productive. Yes, being able to work is a blessing!

Sometimes it is all too much and you are on overload. You may be completely exhausted after spending all night at the hospital with your loved one. You may be so stressed that you feel physically ill. Sometimes you just have to call in sick or ask the boss for a day off. Sometimes a sick day will be enough to help you catch up on sleep and better deal with the demands of giving care. Most bosses understand if you are honest with them about your situation. Tell them if you were sitting up in the emergency room all night and you are so exhausted you might not be able to get much accomplished. Make sure the boss or at least a few co-workers know what you are dealing with. This will help show your veracity and minimize any chance of a co-worker feeling resentful.

Gratitude

Caregivers are thankful for all things great and small. Every day is Thanksgiving Day! Remind yourself of someone you know who is dealing with a worse or more challenging life situation than you are. As bad as things seem, there's always someone who has a worse situation.

Give thanks for what you have. You have an opportunity before you. What? Yes, that's right! If your loved one is suffering with cancer, you have an opportunity to help nurse them back to health or at the least provide comfort at a difficult time in their life. What a wonderful gift of love that is! If your loved one has a terminal prognosis, remember, many people don't have any warning before their loved one passes away. You do. You have time to make it right with them, so you can eliminate any feelings of guilt over wishing you'd have done things differently. You have the gift of time. That is truly something to be thankful for.

Gratitude has a powerful impact on people's lives. Practice it daily. Keep a gratitude journal as a reminder that even though these are tough times, there are some good things happening.

Emotions & Energy

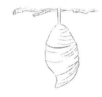

As a caregiver, you deal with a lot of emotions. You deal with your loved one's emotional journey through a serious illness. You deal with his response to that illness. You also deal with his response to you, as a caregiver. By being close to him as his caregiver, you will deal with much more emotion from him than others in his circle of family and friends. You also deal with your own emotions, and the emotions of everyone close to your loved one. You have many feelings come to the surface. You feel badly for what your loved one is going through. You have to deal with his emotions. You may feel some anger at your loved one's illness and the impact it has on his life and yours. You may feel some resentment that you have this new role to play. All these emotions take a toll on the caregiver. You may feel drained of your usual energy at a time when you need it to get through this.

If you have been overdoing it and just aren't up to doing something for your family, communicate that to them. Some families just go on with their usual day-to-day activities because they think that the caregiver appears to be doing just fine. They may assume and expect the caregiver to host holidays and events as done previously. You may need to let them know that as much as you would like to host the holidays this year, you simply aren't able to or that you only could host if you had sufficient help from others.

If you are overdoing it, force yourself to ask for some help and give yourself a break. Don't let the resentment build if no one offers to help. Verbalize the situation. Learn to delegate, before the situation gets too difficult for you.

Conserve your energy for what's important. Dealing with all these emotions can be draining. Suddenly all the little things you used to get uptight about really seem so insignificant compared to what your loved one is going through. You might even feel a little ashamed for your lack of priorities in the past. That's okay. You will come out of this a better person. Forget about the past. Move forward from today.

Start a journal of life lessons from your caregiving journey. What was difficult? What was easier than you thought? What gems did you learn about your loved one? How did your relationship change as you gave care? How have you become a better and stronger person? What are you grateful for each day?

Receiving Love from Others

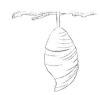

You have been very involved in giving love to the important people in your life. You compassionately care for and show your love for your loved one with cancer. You care for and show your love to your family and friends. You try to keep things "normal" for your family. Often as a caregiver, you try to be everything to everyone.

Your loved one is not the only one who needs to feel love at this time. You, the caregiver, also need to feel the love. If you become too pre-occupied with all the daily activities and demands of caregiving, you may forget to be receptive to the love that others are trying to show you. Receive love from others. Don't get so wrapped up in your caregiver duties, that you unknowingly turn away from love and support offered to you by family and friends. No one expects you to do it all. Sometimes people are reaching out to you and you are so involved with everything going on, you don't even realize it. It can be very uplifting to recognize and feel the love given by others when going through such a difficult and emotional experience. It will encourage you and strengthen you. Use this love to refuel yourself and get through the tough times. Never miss an opportunity to receive love from others. You need their love just as much as your loved one does at this challenging time.

Be open to observing and receiving love from others. It will warm your soul and comfort you. Make a list of things you'd really like to receive or have done. Make a list of what others can help you and your loved one with. Then, when someone asks what they can do for you, you can tell them some loving things they can do to help you. You could even hang the list up in the kitchen and at work for anyone to see.

When someone asks what you'd like for a gift, mention things that will really make a difference for you at this stressful time in your life. Go ahead, be a bit extravagant! It will lift your spirits. It will allow your friends and relatives to be able to do something loving for you. When someone asks what you'd like for a gift, you could mention a gift certificate for a massage, if you are able to get away to use it. This can help caregivers reduce anxiety and depression, if they experience either of those. Perhaps a treat for you would be a carry-in chicken or pizza supper so you don't have to cook one night.

When you are feeling down, what can you do to feel the love from those who are so special in your life? Hug your kids. Hug your grandchildren. Hug your spouse. Hug your parents. Hug your siblings. Hug your closest friends. Hug, hug, and hug! Be willing to accept help from others. Communicate your needs and your caregiver challenges to others. Have a confidant that you can talk openly with about the really tough issues you are dealing with as a caregiver to your loved one.

Be open to receiving love from others in big ways and in small acts of kindness. It will truly help you in getting through some of the tough times. Don't ignore these special gifts. Recognize them for what they are—gifts! Let yourself be encouraged, in knowing that all these helpful people not only care about your loved one, but they also care about you. Finally, don't forget to say thank you to those wonderful people who are remembering you in all those special ways.

Practice Self-Love

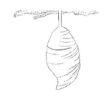

How can you show love to yourself? Tell yourself it's okay to spend a little time relaxing. Tell yourself it's okay to take that nap you have needed for hours, and then do it. Tell yourself it's okay to "cheat" and bring in dinner. It's okay to use paper plates, plastic tableware, and red disposable cups! Remind yourself the house doesn't have to be perfect and immaculate. Sit back, put your feet up, close your eyes, even if only for ten minutes. Meditate your way to better days.

If you are a spiritual person, pray for strength to see you through the challenges that you are facing. Read daily devotions to remind yourself of the comfort of your faith. Read daily inspirational readings for encouragement. Look for a book or calendar that provides daily uplifting messages. Some of these books are written specifically for caregivers. Make it a habit to read those daily messages. Try to pick a time, and as you do this at the same time each day, you will be creating a new habit. Breathe deeply and relax. Practice positive self-talk.

Put on your pajamas, slippers, and most comfortable robe. Fix a cup of tea and curl up on the couch reading or watching TV. Let the ringing phone go to voicemail. Remind yourself that you are a good person and tell yourself why.

Are you housebound? Use your computer to have a mental getaway. With all the things available on the Internet today, you can travel virtually to other lands, listen to music, and listen to talk shows on specific topics. You can find blogs with reading material or watch funny videos.

Buy your favorite magazine and read articles as you can. Magazine articles work great for a quick mental getaway for busy caregivers. They are quick reads and work well when you have little snippets of time available throughout the day and evening. The best part is, you usually can complete an article in one sitting.

Laughter

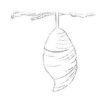

Just as laughter is important for your loved one, it is also important for you, the caregiver. The same benefits your loved one receives from laughter will also be good for you. You will feel good with the flood of endorphins that are released from laughter. You will experience a boost to your immune system, which will be good for your health, given the stress you are under. You will feel more relaxed as a result of laughter. Laughter is good for you emotionally and physically. Yes, it's fun, but it is good medicine and drug-free at that!

You will notice you feel better if you get some laughs in each day. Depending on your loved one's prognosis, this can be very challenging. If your loved one has a bleak prognosis, laughing can be difficult to achieve. Life is certainly serious enough when dealing with cancer. Within reason, try not to take life too seriously.

Laugh out loud. This is no joke! There's professional and non-professional laughter therapy available. Laughter does good things for your body. It has been shown that laughter increases oxygen use. It actually makes you feel better.

Consider keeping your sense of humor and treating yourself to a few laughs as an important component in your self-care program. It is a treat with good side effects.

Watch a comedy. Read a joke book. Visit a funny Internet site. Watch a humorous video. Watch a comedy movie or TV show. Laugh! Listen to the kids' latest jokes. Watch the little kids play. Watch the pets play, tease, and fight. Don't just smile. Let out a good, hearty laugh!

God gives us laughter if we learn to look for it. Sometimes, he even helps us laugh at cancer. I felt rather uncomfortable as I laughed during some of those awkward times. I have my stepmother to thank for helping me to see some of the humor in the situation. I knew if she could laugh, I certainly could as well.

"Is she STILL here?" said my dad as he came out of the bedroom following his afternoon nap. It was so unlike him to be somewhat rude like that. My stepmother and I just had to laugh. I could

have been hurt by that comment, but I knew he wasn't himself. I had driven 130 miles to spend the day with him. I decided to wait until he awoke from his nap before I left to go home. "You didn't think you'd get rid of me that easily did you?" I said to him with a grin.

I never would have thought I could laugh at the cancer that was slowly taking my dad from me. But thank goodness, sometimes laughter is appropriate and a stress-reliever.

My dad had been undergoing some experimental treatments. They were successfully destroying the cancer, but they had taken his voice down to just a whisper. The voice loss was going to be permanent. The experimental drugs were also poisoning his system. He was mentally out of it. Dad had become very weak. He was using a very heavy four-legged cane when he walked. The doctors had to stop the experimental treatment because he couldn't survive it.

As my stepmother and I sat chatting, Dad was in his own little world, paying little to no attention to us. Suddenly, I saw something out of the corner of my eye. In a split-second, Dad had hurled the heavy, four-legged cane directly toward me like a quarterback throwing a fifty-yard touchdown pass. I ducked as it plowed into the couch and nicked my leg. After the initial shock wore off, my stepmother and I laughed. We just never knew what was going to happen next. Was I now going to have to wear a helmet when I came to visit Dad?

Special Treats for Caregivers

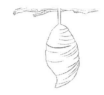

Sometimes you just need to treat yourself to a little something. It doesn't have to be anything significant or costly. Giving yourself a little treat "just because" is good for your soul. Why not? You deserve it. You spend a lot of time caring for your loved one who is battling a difficult disease. Sometimes it's those little things that you do for yourself that serve as a real boost when you could use one. And sometimes, if no one else does it for you, you just have to do it yourself!

After being tied down to caregiving for a period of time, a getaway would be very welcome. You may not be able to get away for a long time, but what about a short mini vacation? You could make it for a couple of hours, overnight, or for a weekend. If you are able to get away longer than that, good for you! Arrange for someone to temporarily take over your caregiver duties until your return.

If your loved one is on hospice, look into respite care. This provides temporary care for your loved one so that you can get some rest and relaxation. This is a beautiful opportunity for caregivers who have little options for getting some relief. You also have the reassurance that your loved one is in good hands.

Buy yourself a bouquet of flowers. They are often inexpensive at discount stores, grocery stores, and gas stations. Watch for flowers reduced in price for quick sale. If you pick a kind that lasts longer, you will more than likely get your money's worth. For example, if you pick reduced-price carnations, rather than lilies, they will probably last much longer. Cut a little off the stem at an angle and use the powder that comes with them to make them last longer.

Treat yourself to a mini spa day…get a cheap or free pedicure. If you have a local beauty college or a hair salon that trains employees you may be able to get a good deal on some pampering.

Sometimes it's a matter of eating a special treat. Go ahead. Once in a while you just have to indulge in some ice cream!

What else could you treat yourself to? This is limited only to your imagination and your wallet. Buy yourself that little something you've been wanting but felt guilty about indulging in.

Spiritual Matters

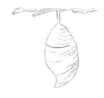

At challenging times like this, you may consider spiritual matters. If you have a spiritual life, maintain and grow your spiritual life. If you have abandoned your spiritual life, now may be the time to rekindle it. Perhaps you have never had a spiritual life, but you are interested now. People often seek one in times of crisis, as they begin to face their mortality as well as that of their loved one.

Lean on your faith, if you have one. Now is not the time to pull away from attending your church services, if you have a church. You need this strength now, more than ever. If you are housebound, listen to services on the radio or TV or Internet. Keep your church body informed of what's going on. They will be a source of support and encouragement for you. Some churches have member care committees. Keep them aware of the latest developments, so they can be a source of support to your loved one.

Read your Bible. Read a daily devotional. Put Post-its with Bible verses around the house to remind yourself of encouraging verses.

Soak up the comfort of your faith. Pray, pray, pray. Ask others to pray for your loved one and yourself. Knowing that others are praying for you and your loved one can be very uplifting.

You may have never been a person of faith. Sometimes the need for a spiritual life first becomes obvious during life's biggest challenges. Your loved one's illness may act as a catalyst causing you to seek a source of comfort. You may feel awkward about taking steps to join a religious group. Sometimes speaking to an acquaintance of faith can be very helpful. They would probably be happy to take you to church and introduce you to the pastor. Look in the Yellow Pages. Search the Internet for religious information. If you decide to visit a church and don't know anyone, usually a member of a welcoming committee will welcome you and lend assistance, if you need any. If you feel like you don't know enough about religion to get started, that's okay. There will be classes to teach you and members of the congregation willing to help you get started on your quest for knowledge.

Self-Love & Avoiding Self-Criticism

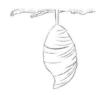

Instead of critiquing yourself over the things you weren't able to do, keep a journal of your journey. Write about what you did do—you'll be amazed at how much you really have done, but forgot about or didn't give yourself credit for. You are an amazing caregiver! Not everyone could do what you do.

It is time to start loving and caring for yourself. It's okay to do and necessary to do. It's time to get help and support. You do not have to go on your journey to caring alone! Think of this as a way of taking care of yourself. Don't try to do it all if you can get any kind of help. Try to involve others from the beginning.

Accept your limitations without being too hard on yourself. It's okay to not be okay! No one expects you to be perfect or a super hero. No one expects you to never get tired, discouraged, or sad. No one expects you to never question why or cry. No one expects you to know all the answers, do all the work, or handle every situation. No one that is, unless you expect that for yourself. Now is not the time to beat yourself up for your shortcomings, which probably aren't as "short" as you think they are. It's okay to feel all those things. It is normal and it is acceptable. You are only human. You have a right to respond to this ugly situation as a human. Feel your feelings, deal with them, and then decide what you can do something about and what you can't.

Take matters into your own hands. That will make you feel empowered. Communicate your feelings to family and friends. Comfort yourself in whatever ways work for you. Forgive yourself for falling short of your expectations. Practice positive self-talk.

Oops, Do You Smell the Litter Box?

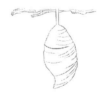

Caregivers give a lot of love. Treat yourself to some regular time with your pet. What a blessing to be loved and comforted by an adoring pet. If you have a pet, don't deny yourself this wonderful comfort at this challenging time in your life.

Take time to smell the roses and Fido or Fluffy! Hug your pet. Pets are so loving and comforting. They will return your love many times over. They sense when you are hurting both physically and emotionally. Let your cat lie on your lap or put its paws around your neck while looking lovingly into your eyes. Let your dog put his head on your lap or lie on your bed or couch by you. Not only will you feel better, but so will Fido and Fluffy.

When you can, be sure to take Fido on his daily walks. Not only will you have a happy dog, you will be doing yourself a favor as well by getting some much-needed exercise. Multi-tasking sometimes works! When you don't have time to walk Fido, make arrangements for someone else to take care of him. This can even be a great job for a neighborhood kid. Cats aren't as forgiving as dogs and are more solitary. They generally demand attention from their owners or their favorite people in the family. I can remember how my cats reacted when I didn't have any "lap time" available for them on some of those busy days. The sad look in their eyes made me feel rather guilty. Remember, they need affection too! Even if you only have a few minutes available for Fluffy, go ahead and indulge her and yourself. It will be good for both of you. And…don't forget to take time to check the litter box! Fluffy will love you even more!

The Little Ones

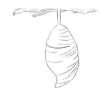

Catch the uplifting feeling of joy from time spent with little ones. Little ones? Yes, young children.

My mother had seven children. She always referred to the youngest children as "The Little Ones." It's a phrase that invokes wonderful memories of my siblings as toddlers and youngsters. There is nothing like the feeling of rocking a baby or toddler as they snuggle against you.

When they aren't sleeping, "The Little Ones" are often very entertaining and can distract you when you are feeling blue. You see life as new and fresh again through the eyes of the little ones.

When life brings hard times, one of the most uplifting comforts is to be with little children who are close to you. Being with children can be such a comfort at the difficult times in life. It certainly reminds us of how tender and precious life is. It reminds us of the innocence of youth and how life goes on despite the difficult days.

The Social Butterfly

Use social media for updates, to express your feelings, and to get help from people.

It may be tempting to avoid social media if you are feeling overwhelmed when dealing with your loved one's illness and all the extra requirements placed on you at this time. This is no time to throw a cover over the computer, your tablet, or your phone. Harness the power of these devices to enlarge your world by reaching out to others. Do not be hesitant to take a break from these devices and social media as you feel a need to. You are in control. You just need to remember that you are in control!

How can you use social media to help you and your loved one? If your loved one is tech-savvy, you have more ways available to provide support to him. The same holds true for you, the caregiver. We have mentioned previously some ways to use email to provide your loved one with inspirational and humorous emails. Here are some ways to use some interactive social media with an impact:

- If your loved one doesn't already have an account, set him up with a social media account. For example, set him up with a Facebook® Account. Help him send out friend requests or ask his friends to send him friend requests.

- You can send him inspirational memes to encourage him when he needs it.

- Update his friends, family, and co-workers on his status when necessary.

- Organize prayer requests for your loved one when he is having difficult days.

- Share pictures of your loved one both past and present.

- Start a social media conversation with friends and family recalling old times and current times. Encourage your loved one to interact with their comments. Even though people may not be able to see him every day, there will be some contact with friends, family, and the outside world. Your loved one will know that others are thinking of him.

- Either you or your loved one could post to social media when he is having a rough day. This usually sparks others to send words of encouragement to him.

- Organize special events for your loved one. Some people have organized a "Celebration of Life" on several occasions for individuals who were alive and fighting cancer. If your loved one is terminal, there is nothing saying you need to wait until he is gone to celebrate his life. It doesn't have to be a surprise. Let your loved one in on the secret. He will have something to look forward to. Ask him who he would like to see, so that you can encourage those individuals to be present. Ask friends to bring food. You probably don't have time to make all the food. Try to have some of your loved one's favorite foods there.

- Let your loved one see you take an active role in fighting his disease. This would have to be an encouragement to him. Send out Facebook® memes supporting research to end his particular kind of cancer. Participate in or support cancer cure fundraisers if possible. (Do not take this on if you feel you are already overburdened. Remember, you must take care of yourself.) If you can't participate, actively advertise the events via social media. It will be uplifting to your loved one to see you participate in a fight against his dreaded disease.

- Organize a visible means of support for your loved one. Select a color and have several t-shirts made in that color with something like "Team Dave" on it. Give these out to friends and family or ask them to purchase these and set some designated times that you all wear them in his presence. Take pictures of people wearing these shirts and post to social media. This visible show of support can be a real encouragement to a loved one.

- Post some of your requests for assistance to social media. Let's say that someone's spouse named Dave has cancer. You could enter a post reading something like this:

  ¤ Some of you have been asking what you can do to help. At this time, we could really use some help with the shopping and the meal preparation. With all the doctor appointments, we are finding it challenging to find time to prepare meals. If you would like to help, here are some things that have tasted good to Dave lately: _____, _____, and _____. If anyone is planning to bring a meal over, please contact _____ to schedule a day and time, so we can spread the meals out.

- Make a point to remember to thank those individuals who are helping you. Yes, you are busy, drained, and perhaps even financially strained. For those who you connect to on social media, you can publically thank them on social media. It will save you time, postage, and phone calls. Seeing that others are contributing may encourage others to take that step as well.

- Sometimes it can feel too emotional and draining for people to speak directly to those who want to support them, yet they still desire that support. Social media can be the "safe" connection, in those cases.

- As the caregiver, you can use social media to let others know how you are doing. There's no need to pretend you are always upbeat and doing great if that is not the truth. Let others know when you need to be lifted up with encouragement and prayers. You will be amazed at the support and encouragement you will receive.

• The beauty of social media is the access twenty-four hours a day to connect to others and to do so silently. When sitting by a hospital bed where your loved one lies sleeping, you can silently post or receive messages. You can vent your anger at the disease or your complete heartbreak at the latest test results. You can share the current status of your loved one. You can share joyous news from the doctors, surgery updates, your loved one's upcoming release date from the hospital, and more. Social media is a powerful tool that can be a blessing to you and your loved one. Just remember, you are in control. When you need to go silent and take a break from it, do so.

It's Okay to Have Feelings and a Life

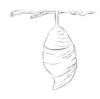

Give yourself permission to have a life. You may not be able to have a "normal" life, depending on the demands of your caregiving. However, you still need to do a few things to try to keep some semblance of being normal. You may have a favorite TV show or want to go to a special social event. You may feel you have to give up everything you desire to be there for your loved one all the time. Recognize your need to have something special to look forward to and do what you can to help make that happen. Think of treating yourself to some of these things as a way of taking care of you. It will help you emotionally and physically if you have something positive to look forward to and enjoy. Think of treating yourself to some time away as part of your medical treatment. It is that important for your well-being!

Love manifests itself in many ways. How many people do you love? How many of those people have you said, "I love you" to? We all love people whom we've never expressed this to. For the cancer caregiver who is already deeply overwhelmed, many expressions could go unnoticed. Your loved one with cancer will sometimes send little signals, which you will want to be receptive to. Friends and relatives will do acts of kindness to help you, some very small, which are easily overlooked. Stay in tune with what is happening around you to realize touching examples of love shown to you. It will warm your heart and lift you up. Often the words escape those we are closest to. Realize that whenever they send you a look or do a kind act, they are sending strong signals of love and concern towards you.

~ Susan Brownell ~

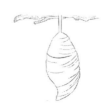

Self-Love also manifests itself in many ways.
If you become totally focused on your loved one, you will lose
yourself and your maximum capacity to care.
If you love them, you must love yourself.
You cannot do for them what you don't do for yourself.

~ Susan Brownell ~

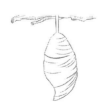

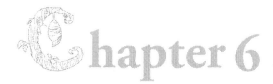

Chapter 6

Hang Glide with the Butterflies!

Everything in life that we really accept undergoes a change. So suffering must become love. That is the mystery.

~ Katherine Mansfield ~

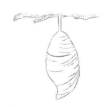

You've emerged from your cocoon of love a changed person.
Make every minute count.
Soar to new heights.
Hang glide with the butterflies!

~ Susan Brownell ~

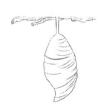

Cocoons are all about change.
Caregiving is about loving, compassionate change.

~ Susan Brownell ~

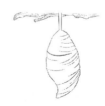

You and your loved one have been going through a process. You've received some upsetting news. You have been processing it and making a lot of decisions. You have come to understand that things are changing. Health issues must be dealt with. Relationships are feeling the impact. You and your loved one are growing and maturing within your cocoons as you really start to gain an understanding of what is happening.

By the time my stepfather became ill with cancer, I knew more about what went on with the loved one and the family and friends of those with cancer. I had learned about the impact of cancer and the caregiving in its various levels of involvement. Although it still wasn't easy, I could handle it better.

I understood that caregiving meant more than just helping the loved one with cancer. It meant helping myself. It also meant helping others deal with the loved one's illness and making relationships endure during times of crisis. Caregiving meant helping others to accept change—change that I first had to accept myself.

When the Butterflies Emerge

When you and your loved one complete the process, you both emerge from your cocoons. You have processed what's happening and you are preparing to take action. You will both be forever changed. You still both have some things in common, but you also both have separate and different priorities. Some of those priorities may be the same as prior to the cancer, and some of those priorities will be different. Each of you must pursue your priorities, and try to get some sense of a normal life again. But, life will not quite be the same. Just as the butterfly is not the same as when it was a caterpillar, so you and your loved one are not the same. There can be good and bad things about change. Forget the negative things. Learn and grow from the good things about this change. Make the decision to accept the change. Love your loved one. Love yourself.

Before, you were looking at life as a caterpillar. You were focused on feeding and constructing your cocoon. The metamorphosis that goes on inside the cocoon brings change to you and your loved one.

Did you know that butterflies have compound eyes? They are among the creatures with the best vision. They can see things that we can't. They can see ultraviolet light. They use this to help them find the nectar that sustains them. Cancer patients and their caregivers need compound eyes. They need to have that high-powered vision to understand what is happening.

In time, your loved one and you will emerge from your cocoons. You will both be changed forever.

You will forever carry the experience of being a caregiver to someone facing a serious illness. You will see and experience things that you wouldn't have if your loved one had been well. You will learn about life, fear, courage, strength, and perhaps even about death.

Your loved one also will never be the same. If your loved one is a survivor, how will his role change? If your loved one does not survive, how will your life change? Either way, there will be a big change when the cocoon is empty. This could mean the butterfly is alive and well. This could also mean the butterfly has left us and moved on to another place. The empty cocoon symbolizes a major lifetime change.

Caregivers who are suddenly done with their caregiver duties often experience a range of emotions. They may feel a great sense of relief. They may feel great sadness if their loved one didn't survive. They may feel an emptiness. After all the busy and demanding days, they may suddenly have a lot of free time available. That should be a good feeling, right? This is not always the case with caregivers. All of a sudden, they are not needed anymore. In an instant, they are free to go back to their "normal" life, whatever that is. Although it may be a relief, this can take some adjustment.

How do you cope with these changes? After depriving yourself of social events, shopping, and many other things for a long period of time, a caregiver may have to make a bit of an effort to get out there again socially. Eventually, you will find joy again.

As you begin to deal with your new life, take some time to renew yourself. You have been through a lot. You may not even realize how much you have been through until this is long over. Give yourself some of those special treats and get a lot of rest. Try to get back on track with your diet and exercise if you got off schedule while you were giving care. Start seeing people that you didn't have time to connect with before. As you begin to transition back to your "normal" life, do it with self-love. Don't put pressure on yourself. Do things as you are ready to. Just keep moving forward…with love.

Releasing the Silk Threads

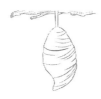

How do you cope with the change produced by your loved one's transition? As a caregiver you may be over-protective because of what your loved one has gone through. At the same time, he deserves to resume living on his terms. When his health and strength improves, he wants and needs to get back to a more normal life. Sometimes as an involved caregiver, it can be difficult to let go. Remember that you cared for your loved one, in love, at a time when he needed you. Now, you must gently loosen your hold on those golden threads of love that encased his cocoon. Now, you must let him go. Let him fly free. Do it with love.

Just as you have to adjust to a new life after the cocoon, so does your loved one. Cancer survivors have to pick up the pieces and move on with life. Will things be the same? Will your loved one have changed? Survivors of cancer remain impacted by the disease. There are fears and concerns about the biannual checkups. The dread of a reoccurrence is often in the back of their mind. Just like you, your loved one will look at life differently after this experience. But he will learn to live his life with gratitude for each new day. He will find joy once again. He will do it all with love.

If your loved one does not survive, you must also let him go. You will have to adapt to this new life with the void of a very special person. You know that you will always have the memories, but that's not enough when you are grieving. You will take whatever time you need to accept and deal with your new life. You may need to attend a grief support group. Lean on your faith and friends as you release the silk threads.

Living Your Best Butterfly Life

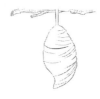

Life is short. You want to make wise use of the time given. Life is fragile. Do you know how long a butterfly lives? Some are destined to live as few as forty-eight hours, some for two weeks. Others, such as monarch butterflies, live up to nine months. That's the best-case scenario! Some butterflies, such as the monarch, migrate to Mexico. Imagine the obstacles in the way of these fragile creatures as they make a journey like that.

Butterflies have undergone a tremendous change through their metamorphoses. As they emerge from their cocoon, they are very delicate. Their wings are wet and shouldn't be touched as they are drying. Their wings are very important to their well-being. Their wings are also fragile, and the oils from human skin can cause damage to them.

Everyone wants to be near a butterfly. The butterfly projects love, beauty, goodness, happiness. It is well-known that butterflies do not live very long lives. Yet, in some religions, they symbolize eternal life. Whenever you speak to older folks, they often tell you that the older they get, the quicker the years go by. Do you think the same concept holds true for caterpillars turned butterflies? Even though some butterflies live only a few days, while others live long enough to make the long migration to Mexico, butterflies appear so full of life and so joyful. It is as though they evoke love and happiness wherever they go. Could it be? Have they learned to live life to the fullest regardless of what is happening to them and what is happening around them?

Yes, life is fragile. But life is love. And love is bigger than life. Spread the love to your loved one and yourself. Accept the love offered to you in little ways and big ways. Emerging from the cocoon, you and your loved one have new things and emotions to experience. You have both changed. As much as you'd like to, you know you aren't supposed to touch a butterfly's wings. Stand still. Look at your loved one's empty cocoon. Marvel at this miracle of transformation. Take in the beauty. Become aware of your senses in a new way. Feel the love as the butterfly swoops past your face, in a teasing way. Catch your breath as the butterfly's wings almost brush against your cheek! Catch your breath as you touch understanding.

Acknowledgements

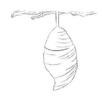

Cocoon Interior Illustrations rights belong to the author.
Cover Illustration by: Dima Kasovski
Cover Illustration rights belong to the author

With love and heartfelt thanks to some special people in my life:

My husband, my rock, for his support and encouragement. My children and grandchildren, daughter in-law and son-in-law for their understanding of my "absence" over an extended period while I was writing.

References

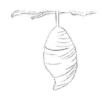

The quotations by Elisabeth Kubler-Ross are used with the permission of the Elizabeth Kubler-Ross Foundation.

The quotation by Katherine Mansfield is used with the permission of the Katherine Mansfield Society in New Zealand.

About the Author

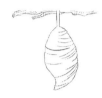

Susan Brownell is the founder of a website for caregivers. It is SanctuaryForCancerCaregivers.com. Over a consecutive eight-year period, her mother, father, stepmother, and stepfather were diagnosed with cancer. One by one they were diagnosed. One by one they left this earth. Susan has also helped care for other aging and sick relatives. Susan struggled with the stress and exhaustion of caregiving. She knows the pain and the heartbreak. She knows the physical and emotional toll caregiving takes. Susan believes every caregiver could use a healthy dose of encouragement and inspiration to get them through the tough times.

Susan has authored another book in the Cocoon of Love series. It is called, *Cocoon of Love for Caregivers: 365 Inspirational Readings for Busy Caregivers.*

A third book Susan has written for caregivers is called, *51 Secrets Every Cancer Caregiver Needs to Know.*

Susan also writes children's books. She likes to focus on fun stories with a lesson for children. She will soon be releasing two children's books.

Besides writing, one of Susan's passions is to help cancer caregivers with their daily struggles. She wishes she would have had some help available when she was starting her role as a caregiver.

Watch her websites for information on upcoming books and other information to help caregivers.

To keep up with the latest from Susan, visit her websites, YouTube Channel, or follow her on social media:

susanbrownell.com
sanctuaryforcancercaregivers.com
Twitter: @SusanBrownell
Facebook: Search for "Sanctuary For Cancer Caregivers"

Made in the USA
San Bernardino, CA
11 December 2019